BLACKWELL'S
UNDERGROUND CLINICAL VIGNETTES

PATHOPHYSIOLOGY
VOL. I, 3E

BLACKWELL'S
UNDERGROUND CLINICAL VIGNETTES

PATHOPHYSIOLOGY VOL. I, 3E

VIKAS BHUSHAN, MD
University of California, San Francisco, Class of 1991
Series Editor, Diagnostic Radiologist

VISHAL PALL, MBBS
Government Medical College, Chandigarh, India, Class of 1996
Series Editor, U. of Texas, Galveston, Resident in Internal Medicine &
Preventive Medicine

TAO LE, MD
University of California, San Francisco, Class of 1996

HOANG NGUYEN, MD, MBA
Northwestern University, Class of 2001

VIPAL SONI, MD
UCLA School of Medicine, Class of 1999

Blackwell
Science

CONTRIBUTORS

Robert Nason
University of Texas Medical Branch, Class of 2003

Tisha Wang
University of Texas Medical Branch, Class of 2002

Kristen Lem Mygdal, MD
University of Kansas School of Medicine, Resident in Radiology

Fadi Abu Shahin, MD
University of Damascus, Syria, Class of 1999

Jose M. Fierro, MD
La Salle University, Mexico City

© 2002 by Blackwell Science, Inc.

Editorial Offices:

Commerce Place, 350 Main Street, Malden,
    Massachusetts 02148, USA
Osney Mead, Oxford OX2 0EL, England
25 John Street, London WC1N 2BS, England
23 Ainslie Place, Edinburgh EH3 6AJ, Scotland
54 University Street, Carlton, Victoria 3053,
    Australia

Other Editorial Offices:

Blackwell Wissenschafts-Verlag GmbH,
    Kurfürstendamm 57, 10707 Berlin, Germany
Blackwell Science KK, MG Kodenmacho Building,
    7-10 Kodenmacho Nihombashi, Chuo-ku,
    Tokyo 104, Japan
Iowa State University Press, A Blackwell Science
    Company, 2121 S. State Avenue, Ames, Iowa
    50014-8300, USA

Acquisitions: Laura DeYoung
Development: Amy Nuttbrock
Production: Lorna Hind and Shawn Girsberger
Manufacturing: Lisa Flanagan
Marketing Manager: Kathleen Mulcahy
Cover design by Leslie Haimes
Interior design by Shawn Girsberger
Typeset by TechBooks
Printed and bound by Capital City Press

Blackwell's Underground Clinical Vignettes:
    Pathophysiology I, 3e
ISBN 0-632-04551-5

Printed in the United States of America
02 03 04 05 5 4 3 2 1

First Indian Reprint 2002

Printed and bound by Multivista Global Limited,
Chennai - 600 042.

The Blackwell Science logo is a trade mark of
Blackwell Science Ltd., registered at the United
Kingdom Trade Marks Registry

Library of Congress Cataloging-in-Publication Data
Bhushan, Vikas.
Blackwell's underground clinical vignettes.
Pathophysiology / author, Vikas Bhushan. – 3rd ed.
    p. ; cm. – (Underground clinical vignettes)
Rev. ed. of: Pathophysiology / Vikas Bhushan.
2nd ed. c1999. ISBN 0-632-04551-5 (pbk.)
1. Physiology, Pathological – Case studies.
2. Physicians – Licenses – United States –
Examinations – Study guides.
    [DNLM: 1. Clinical Medicine – Case Report.
2. Clinical Medicine – Problems and Exercises. WB
18.2 B575bb 2002] I. Title: Underground clinical
vignettes. Pathophysiology. II. Pathophysiology.
III. Title. IV. Series.
    RB113 .B459 2002
    616.07'076–dc21

2001004931

CONTENTS

ACKNOWLEDGMENTS

Throughout the production of this book, we have had the support of many friends and colleagues. Special thanks to our support team including Anu Gupta, Andrea Fellows, Anastasia Anderson, Srishti Gupta, Mona Pall, Jonathan Kirsch and Chirag Amin. For prior contributions we thank Gianni Le Nguyen, Tarun Mathur, Alex Grimm, Sonia Santos and Elizabeth Sanders.

We have enjoyed working with a world-class international publishing group at Blackwell Science, including Laura DeYoung, Amy Nuttbrock, Lisa Flanagan, Shawn Girsberger, Lorna Hind and Gordon Tibbitts. For help with securing images for the entire series we also thank Lee Martin, Kristopher Jones, Tina Panizzi and Peter Anderson at the University of Alabama, the Armed Forces Institute of Pathology, and many of our fellow Blackwell Science authors.

For submitting comments, corrections, editing, proofreading, and assistance across all of the vignette titles in all editions, we collectively thank:

Tara Adamovich, Carolyn Alexander, Kris Alden, Henry E. Aryan, Lynman Bacolor, Natalie Barteneva, Dean Bartholomew, Debashish Behera, Sumit Bhatia, Sanjay Bindra, Dave Brinton, Julianne Brown, Alexander Brownie, Tamara Callahan, David Canes, Bryan Casey, Aaron Caughey, Hebert Chen, Jonathan Cheng, Arnold Cheung, Arnold Chin, Simion Chiosea, Yoon Cho, Samuel Chung, Gretchen Conant, Vladimir Coric, Christopher Cosgrove, Ronald Cowan, Karekin R. Cunningham, A. Sean Dalley, Rama Dandamudi, Sunit Das, Ryan Armando Dave, John David, Emmanuel de la Cruz, Robert DeMello, Navneet Dhillon, Sharmila Dissanaike, David Donson, Adolf Etchegaray, Alea Eusebio, Priscilla A. Frase, David Frenz, Kristin Gaumer, Yohannes Gebreegziabher, Anil Gehi, Tony George, L.M. Gotanco, Parul Goyal, Alex Grimm, Rajeev Gupta, Ahmad Halim, Sue Hall, David Hasselbacher, Tamra Heimert, Michelle Higley, Dan Hoit, Eric Jackson, Tim Jackson, Sundar Jayaraman, Pei-Ni Jone, Aarchan Joshi, Rajni K. Jutla, Faiyaz Kapadi, Seth Karp, Aaron S. Kesselheim, Sana Khan, Andrew Pin-wei Ko, Francis Kong, Paul Konitzky, Warren S. Krackov, Benjamin H.S. Lau, Ann LaCasce, Connie Lee, Scott Lee, Guillermo Lehmann, Kevin Leung, Paul Levett, Warren Levinson, Eric Ley, Ken Lin,

Pavel Lobanov, J. Mark Maddox, Aram Mardian, Samir Mehta, Gil Melmed, Joe Messina, Robert Mosca, Michael Murphy, Vivek Nandkarni, Siva Naraynan, Carvell Nguyen, Linh Nguyen, Deanna Nobleza, Craig Nodurft, George Noumi, Darin T. Okuda, Adam L. Palance, Paul Pamphrus, Jinha Park, Sonny Patel, Ricardo Pietrobon, Riva L. Rahl, Aashita Randeria, Rachan Reddy, Beatriu Reig, Marilou Reyes, Jeremy Richmon, Tai Roe, Rick Roller, Rajiv Roy, Diego Ruiz, Anthony Russell, Sanjay Sahgal, Urmimala Sarkar, John Schilling, Isabell Schmitt, Daren Schuhmacher, Sonal Shah, Fadi Abu Shahin, Mae Sheikh-Ali, Edie Shen, Justin Smith, John Stulak, Lillian Su, Julie Sundaram, Rita Suri, Seth Sweetser, Antonio Talayero, Merita Tan, Mark Tanaka, Eric Taylor, Jess Thompson, Indi Trehan, Raymond Turner, Okafo Uchenna, Eric Uyguanco, Richa Varma, John Wages, Alan Wang, Eunice Wang, Andy Weiss, Amy Williams, Brian Yang, Hany Zaky, Ashraf Zaman and David Zipf.

For generously contributing images to the entire *Underground Clinical Vignette* Step 1 series, we collectively thank the staff at Blackwell Science in Oxford, Boston, and Berlin as well as:

- Axford, J. *Medicine.* Osney Mead: Blackwell Science Ltd, 1996. Figures 2.14, 2.15, 2.16, 2.27, 2.28, 2.31, 2.35, 2.36, 2.38, 2.43, 2.65a, 2.65b, 2.65c, 2.103b, 2.105b, 3.20b, 3.21, 8.27, 8.27b, 8.77b, 8.77c, 10.81b, 10.96a, 12.28a, 14.6, 14.16, 14.50.

- Bannister B, Begg N, Gillespie S. *Infectious Disease, 2ⁿᵈ Edition.* Osney Mead: Blackwell Science Ltd, 2000. Figures 2.8, 3.4, 5.28, 18.10, W5.32, W5.6.

- Berg D. *Advanced Clinical Skills and Physical Diagnosis.* Blackwell Science Ltd., 1999. Figures 7.10, 7.12, 7.13, 7.2, 7.3, 7.7, 7.8, 7.9, 8.1, 8.2, 8.4, 8.5, 9.2, 10.2, 11.3, 11.5, 12.6.

- Cuschieri A, Hennessy TPJ, Greenhalgh RM, Rowley DA, Grace PA. *Clinical Surgery.* Osney Mead: Blackwell Science Ltd, 1996. Figures 13.19, 18.22, 18.33.

- Gillespie SH, Bamford K. *Medical Microbiology and Infection at a Glance.* Osney Mead: Blackwell Science Ltd, 2000. Figures 20, 23.

- Ginsberg L. *Lecture Notes on Neurology, 7ᵗʰ Edition.* Osney Mead: Blackwell Science Ltd, 1999. Figures 12.3, 18.3, 18.3b.

- Elliott T, Hastings M, Desselberger U. *Lecture Notes on Medical Microbiology, 3ʳᵈ Edition.* Osney Mead: Blackwell Science Ltd, 1997. Figures 2, 5, 7, 8, 9, 11, 12, 14, 15, 16, 17, 19, 20, 25, 26, 27, 29, 30, 34, 35, 52.

- Mehta AB, Hoffbrand AV. *Haematology at a Glance.* Osney Mead: Blackwell Science Ltd, 2000. Figures 22.1, 22.2, 22.3.

Please let us know if your name has been missed or misspelled and we will be happy to make the update in the next edition.

PREFACE TO THE 3RD EDITION

We were very pleased with the overwhelmingly positive student feedback for the 2nd edition of our *Underground Clinical Vignettes* series. Well over 100,000 copies of the UCV books are in print and have been used by students all over the world.

Over the last two years we have accumulated and incorporated **over a thousand "updates"** and improvements suggested by you, our readers, including:

- many additions of specific boards and wards testable content

- deletions of redundant and overlapping cases

- reordering and reorganization of all cases in both series

- a new master index by case name in each Atlas

- correction of a few factual errors

- diagnosis and treatment updates

- addition of 5–20 new cases in every book

- and the addition of clinical exam photographs within *UCV— Anatomy*

And most important of all, the third edition sets now include two brand new **COLOR ATLAS** supplements, one for each Clinical Vignette series.

- The *UCV–Basic Science Color Atlas* (*Step 1*) includes over 250 color plates, divided into gross pathology, microscopic pathology (histology), hematology, and microbiology (smears).

- The *UCV–Clinical Science Color Atlas* (*Step 2*) has over 125 color plates, including patient images, dermatology, and funduscopy.

Each atlas image is descriptively captioned and linked to its corresponding Step 1 case, Step 2 case, and/or Step 2 MiniCase.

How Atlas Links Work:

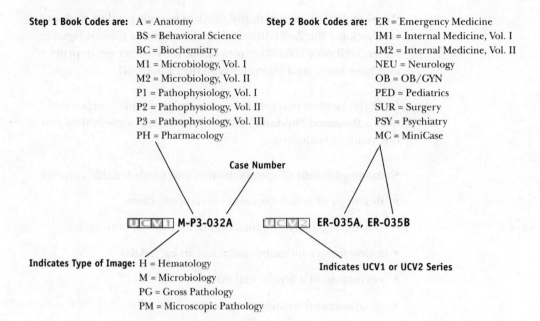

Step 1 Book Codes are:
A = Anatomy
BS = Behavioral Science
BC = Biochemistry
M1 = Microbiology, Vol. I
M2 = Microbiology, Vol. II
P1 = Pathophysiology, Vol. I
P2 = Pathophysiology, Vol. II
P3 = Pathophysiology, Vol. III
PH = Pharmacology

Step 2 Book Codes are:
ER = Emergency Medicine
IM1 = Internal Medicine, Vol. I
IM2 = Internal Medicine, Vol. II
NEU = Neurology
OB = OB/GYN
PED = Pediatrics
SUR = Surgery
PSY = Psychiatry
MC = MiniCase

Case Number

UCV1 M-P3-032A   UCV2 ER-035A, ER-035B

Indicates Type of Image:
H = Hematology
M = Microbiology
PG = Gross Pathology
PM = Microscopic Pathology

Indicates UCV1 or UCV2 Series

- If the Case number (032, 035, etc.) is not followed by a letter, then there is only one image. Otherwise A, B, C, D indicate up to 4 images.

Bold Faced Links: In order to give you access to the largest number of images possible, we have chosen to cross link the Step 1 and 2 series.

- If the link is bold-faced this indicates that the link is direct (i.e, Step 1 Case with the Basic Science Step 1 Atlas link).

- If the link is not bold-faced this indicates that the link is indirect (Step 1 case with Clinical Science Step 2 Atlas link or vice versa).

We have also implemented a few structural changes upon your request:

- Each current and future edition of our popular *First Aid for the USMLE Step 1* (Appleton & Lange/McGraw-Hill) and *First Aid for the USMLE Step 2* (Appleton & Lange/McGraw-Hill) book will be linked to the corresponding UCV case.

- We eliminated UCV → First Aid links as they frequently become out of date, as the *First Aid* books are revised yearly.

- The Color Atlas is also specially designed for quizzing—captions are descriptive and do not give away the case name directly.

We hope the updated UCV series will remain a unique and well-integrated study tool that provides compact clinical correlations to basic science information. They are designed to be easy and fun (comparatively) to read, and helpful for both licensing exams and the wards.

We invite your corrections and suggestions for the fourth edition of these books. For the first submission of each factual correction or new vignette that is selected for inclusion in the fourth edition, you will receive a personal acknowledgment in the revised book. If you submit over 20 high-quality corrections, additions or new vignettes we will also consider **inviting you to become a "Contributor" on the book of your choice**. If you are interested in becoming a potential "Contributor" or "Author" on a future UCV book, or working with our team in developing additional books, please also e-mail us your CV/resume.

We prefer that you submit corrections or suggestions via electronic mail to **UCVteam@yahoo.com**. Please include "Underground Vignettes" as the subject of your message. If you do not have access to e-mail, use the following mailing address: Blackwell Publishing, Attn: UCV Editors, 350 Main Street, Malden, MA 02148, USA.

Vikas Bhushan
Vishal Pall
Tao Le
October 2001

HOW TO USE THIS BOOK

This series was originally developed to address the increasing number of clinical vignette questions on medical examinations, including the USMLE Step 1 and Step 2. It is also designed to supplement and complement the popular *First Aid for the USMLE Step 1* (Appleton & Lange/McGraw Hill) and *First Aid for the USMLE Step 2* (Appleton & Lange/McGraw Hill).

Each UCV 1 book uses a series of approximately 100 **"supra-prototypical" cases as a way to condense testable facts and associations**. The clinical vignettes in this series are designed to incorporate as many testable facts as possible into a cohesive and memorable clinical picture. The vignettes represent composites drawn from general and specialty textbooks, reference books, thousands of USMLE style questions and the personal experience of the authors and reviewers.

Although each case tends to present all the signs, symptoms, and diagnostic findings for a particular illness, **patients generally will not present with such a "complete" picture either clinically or on a medical examination**. Cases are not meant to simulate a potential real patient or an exam vignette. All the **boldfaced "buzzwords" are for learning purposes** and are not necessarily expected to be found in any one patient with the disease.

Definitions of selected important terms are placed within the vignettes in (SMALL CAPS) in parentheses. Other parenthetical remarks often refer to the pathophysiology or mechanism of disease. The format should also help students learn to present cases succinctly during oral "bullet" presentations on clinical rotations. The cases are meant to serve as a condensed review, not as a primary reference. The information provided in this book has been prepared with a great deal of thought and careful research. This book should not, however, be considered as your sole source of information. Corrections, suggestions and submissions of new cases are encouraged and will be acknowledged and incorporated when appropriate in future editions.

ABBREVIATIONS

5-ASA	5-aminosalicylic acid
ABGs	arterial blood gases
ABVD	adriamycin/bleomycin/vincristine/dacarbazine
ACE	angiotensin-converting enzyme
ACTH	adrenocorticotropic hormone
ADH	antidiuretic hormone
AFP	alpha fetal protein
AI	aortic insufficiency
AIDS	acquired immunodeficiency syndrome
ALL	acute lymphocytic leukemia
ALT	alanine transaminase
AML	acute myelogenous leukemia
ANA	antinuclear antibody
ARDS	adult respiratory distress syndrome
ASD	atrial septal defect
ASO	anti-streptolysin O
AST	aspartate transaminase
AV	arteriovenous
BE	barium enema
BP	blood pressure
BUN	blood urea nitrogen
CAD	coronary artery disease
CALLA	common acute lymphoblastic leukemia antigen
CBC	complete blood count
CHF	congestive heart failure
CK	creatine kinase
CLL	chronic lymphocytic leukemia
CML	chronic myelogenous leukemia
CMV	cytomegalovirus
CNS	central nervous system
COPD	chronic obstructive pulmonary disease
CPK	creatine phosphokinase
CSF	cerebrospinal fluid
CT	computed tomography
CVA	cerebrovascular accident
CXR	chest x-ray
DIC	disseminated intravascular coagulation
DIP	distal interphalangeal
DKA	diabetic ketoacidosis
DM	diabetes mellitus
DTRs	deep tendon reflexes
DVT	deep venous thrombosis

EBV	Epstein–Barr virus
ECG	electrocardiography
Echo	echocardiography
EF	ejection fraction
EGD	esophagogastroduodenoscopy
EMG	electromyography
ERCP	endoscopic retrograde cholangiopancreatography
ESR	erythrocyte sedimentation rate
FEV	forced expiratory volume
FNA	fine needle aspiration
FTA-ABS	fluorescent treponemal antibody absorption
FVC	forced vital capacity
GFR	glomerular filtration rate
GH	growth hormone
GI	gastrointestinal
GM-CSF	granulocyte macrophage colony stimulating factor
GU	genitourinary
HAV	hepatitis A virus
hcG	human chorionic gonadotrophin
HEENT	head, eyes, ears, nose, and throat
HIV	human immunodeficiency virus
HLA	human leukocyte antigen
HPI	history of present illness
HR	heart rate
HRIG	human rabies immune globulin
HS	hereditary spherocytosis
ID/CC	identification and chief complaint
IDDM	insulin-dependent diabetes mellitus
Ig	immunoglobulin
IGF	insulin-like growth factor
IM	intramuscular
JVP	jugular venous pressure
KUB	kidneys/ureter/bladder
LDH	lactate dehydrogenase
LES	lower esophageal sphincter
LFTs	liver function tests
LP	lumbar puncture
LV	left ventricular
LVH	left ventricular hypertrophy
Lytes	electrolytes
MCHC	mean corpuscular hemoglobin concentration
MCV	mean corpuscular volume
MEN	multiple endocrine neoplasia

MGUS	monoclonal gammopathy of undetermined significance
MHC	major histocompatibility complex
MI	myocardial infarction
MOPP	mechlorethamine/vincristine (Oncovorin)/procarbazine/prednisone
MR	magnetic resonance (imaging)
NHL	non-Hodgkin's lymphoma
NIDDM	non-insulin-dependent diabetes mellitus
NPO	nil per os (nothing by mouth)
NSAID	nonsteroidal anti-inflammatory drug
PA	posteroanterior
PIP	proximal interphalangeal
PBS	peripheral blood smear
PE	physical exam
PFTs	pulmonary function tests
PMI	point of maximal intensity
PMN	polymorphonuclear leukocyte
PT	prothrombin time
PTCA	percutaneous transluminal angioplasty
PTH	parathyroid hormone
PTT	partial thromboplastin time
PUD	peptic ulcer disease
RBC	red blood cell
RPR	rapid plasma reagin
RR	respiratory rate
RS	Reed–Sternberg (cell)
RV	right ventricular
RVH	right ventricular hypertrophy
SBFT	small bowel follow-through
SIADH	syndrome of inappropriate secretion of ADH
SLE	systemic lupus erythematosus
STD	sexually transmitted disease
TFTs	thyroid function tests
tPA	tissue plasminogen activator
TSH	thyroid-stimulating hormone
TIBC	total iron-binding capacity
TIPS	transjugular intrahepatic portosystemic shunt
TPO	thyroid peroxidase
TSH	thyroid-stimulating hormone
TTP	thrombotic thrombocytopenic purpura
UA	urinalysis
UGI	upper GI
US	ultrasound

ID/CC   A 48-year-old **male** with a history of **hypertension** is brought by ambulance to the emergency room because of the development of **sudden sharp, tearing, intractable left chest pain with radiation to the back**.

HPI   When he first arrives, he shows a declining level of consciousness, becomes **pale** and **short of breath** (DYSPNEA), has **decreased urine output** (OLIGURIA), and is unable to move his left arm and leg; subsequently he **faints** (SYNCOPE).

PE   VS: **marked hypotension** (BP 90/50) in left arm, with significantly higher reading in right arm (BP 170/80). PE: **pallor; cyanosis; diaphoresis**; indistinct heart sounds; **aortic regurgitation murmur** (high-pitched, blowing, diastolic decrescendo murmur); inspiratory crackles at lung bases bilaterally (due to pulmonary edema); **anuria** (due to decreased renal perfusion); **left-sided hemiplegia**.

Labs   ECG: no evidence of myocardial infarct.

Imaging   CT/MR: **spiraling intimal flap with true and false lumen** (DOUBLE-BARREL AORTA). Angio, aortography: confirmatory. CXR: **mediastinal widening** (due to hemorrhage).

Gross Pathology   Longitudinal separation of tunica media of aortic wall.

Treatment   ICU monitoring for shock; antihypertensive agents to decrease vascular shear forces (avoid arteriolar dilators such as hydralazine); surgical correction.

Discussion   Aortic dissection is a **life-threatening** condition requiring immediate treatment. Predisposing factors include **hypertension** and connective tissue diseases (cystic medial degeneration as in Marfan's syndrome); complications include rupture and extension. **Sudden death** may occur with **pericardial tamponade** or **extension of dissection into coronary arteries**.

Atlas Links   🄄🄒🅅🄀 PG-P1-001, PM-P1-001

ID/CC A 31-year-old white male who was diagnosed with **Marfan's syndrome** more than 20 years ago **recently** developed **severe shortness of breath**.

HPI He denies smoking or drinking and claims to have had no major illnesses in the past.

PE VS: **pulse bounding, large in volume, and collapsing** (WATER-HAMMER OR CORRIGAN'S PULSE), producing **wide pulse pressure** with rapid rise and fall. PE: soft, high-pitched, blowing **diastolic decrescendo murmur heard best at left sternal border** with patient leaning forward and in expiration; diastolic murmur heard when femoral artery compressed with stethoscope (DUROZIEZ' SIGN).

Labs ECG: left ventricular hypertrophy (LVH).

Imaging CXR: left ventricular dilatation. Echo: LVH; Doppler confirmatory.

Gross Pathology Caused by defect of aortic valves or roots that leads to regurgitation of blood from aorta into left ventricle.

Treatment Surgical **prosthetic valve replacement** for symptomatic patients or for asymptomatic patients with LV dysfunction. For symptomatic patients with normal LV function, diuretics or afterload-reducing drugs may be beneficial. Antibiotic prophylaxis against infective endocarditis before undergoing surgical or dental procedures.

Discussion Common causes of aortic insufficiency include congenital bicuspid valve, infective endocarditis, and hypertension; less common causes include rheumatic heart disease and aortic root diseases (e.g., Marfan's syndrome, ankylosing spondylitis, Reiter's syndrome, tertiary syphilis).

ID/CC A **24-year-old** man complains of easy fatigability, dyspnea on mild exertion, and **angina**.

HPI He also admits to having occasional spells of **lightheadedness** and **fainting** while playing basketball.

PE **Crescendo-decrescendo systolic ejection murmur to right of sternum and radiating to neck**; soft S2 with **paradoxical splitting** (due to pulmonary valve closure preceding aortic valve closure); weak and delayed ("parvus et tardus") carotid pulses.

Labs ECG: left ventricular hypertrophy.

Imaging CXR: calcifications on valve leaflets and enlarged cardiac shadow (due to large left ventricle). Echo: presence of bicuspid aortic valve.

Gross Pathology Congenital bicuspid valve with calcification.

Treatment Balloon valvuloplasty; surgical prosthetic replacement or changing of normal pulmonary valve to aortic site and insertion of pulmonary prosthesis (ROSS PROCEDURE); antibiotic prophylaxis with penicillin prior to surgical or dental procedures.

Discussion Causes of aortic stenosis include **congenital bicuspid aortic valve** (more common in males), **progressive degenerative calcification** of normal valves (more common in elderly males), and rheumatic heart disease (the mitral valve is also involved in 95% of individuals with rheumatic disease of the aortic valve).

Atlas Link UCV1 PG-P1-003

ID/CC	A 59-year-old white male complains of **pain in the calf muscles** during exercise (CLAUDICATION) along with coldness and numbness in both legs; his symptoms have been occurring for a year and are **relieved by rest**.
HPI	The patient has also been **impotent** and has been experiencing abdominal pain (due to mesenteric ischemia) about half an hour after eating (POSTPRANDIAL PAIN). He **smokes** two packs of cigarettes a day.
PE	VS: **hypertension** (BP 150/100). PE: **diminished peripheral pulses** bilaterally; **loss of hair** over dorsum of feet and hands; decreased temperature in hands and feet; **carotid and femoral arterial bruits**; atrophy of calf muscles.
Labs	**Elevated LDL and decreased HDL**; elevated total serum cholesterol.
Imaging	Angio: multiple large **atheromatous plaques in aortoiliac distribution**. XR, plain: irregular arterial vascular calcifications. US, Doppler: high-velocity poststenotic flow jet.
Gross Pathology	Early: fatty streak in subendothelium; late: **fibrofatty plaque** formation with dystrophic calcification (atheroma) with narrowing of lumen of vessel wall.
Micro Pathology	Early: **foam cells** with intimal proliferation of smooth muscle cells; late: smooth muscle cells synthesize collagen and form **fibrous cap** with **necrotic lipid core** and fibrous plaque.
Treatment	Exercise; smoking cessation; low-dose aspirin; control of hypertension; cholesterol-lowering drugs (e.g., lovastatin); angioplasty; coronary stenting; coronary artery bypass grafting (CABG).
Discussion	Atherosclerosis is the main cause of coronary artery disease and the leading cause of mortality in the United States. Plaques are commonly found in the abdominal aorta, coronary arteries, popliteal arteries, descending thoracic aorta, internal carotid arteries, and circle of Willis arteries. Thus, they are responsible for aortic aneurysms, CAD, peripheral vascular disease, intestinal angina, renovascular hypertension, and cerebrovascular disease.
Atlas Links	UCV1 PG-P1-004A, PG-P1-004B, PM-P1-004A, PM-P1-004B

ID/CC A 47-year-old man complains of occasional **palpitations** and **shortness of breath**.

HPI He also says that he occasionally experiences mild **dizziness** and chest discomfort.

PE VS: **irregularly irregular** pulse. PE: loss of a waves in jugular venous pulse; variable-intensity S1 with occasional S3.

Labs ECG: variable ventricular rate (80 to 200); can be > 200 with wide QRS if associated with accessory pathway; **no discernible P waves seen**. Normal CK-MB.

Imaging CXR: normal. Echo: enlarged left atrium.

Treatment **Beta-blockers; calcium channel blockers; digitalis** (to decrease conduction at AV node in order to prevent ventricular arrhythmias); chemical cardioversion with **class IA, IC, or III antiarrhythmics** to convert back to sinus rhythm if patient remains symptomatic; **electrical cardioversion** (if associated with ventricular tachycardia); patients should also be **anticoagulated** with warfarin to prevent embolic disease.

Discussion Atrial fibrillation, the most common chronic arrhythmia, is associated with a high risk of **embolic disease**. Causes include drugs, mitral valve disease, hypertensive and ischemic heart disease, dilated cardiomyopathy, alcoholism, **hyperthyroidism**, pericarditis, pulmonary embolism, exercise, atrial septal defect, chronic lung disease, and cardiac surgery. It may also be idiopathic.

ID/CC	A **50-year-old woman** complains of recurrent, **transient losses of consciousness** (SYNCOPE) and **dizziness**.
HPI	For the past few months she has had continuous mild to moderate **fever, fatigue, sweating, and joint pains** (ARTHRALGIAS) and has experienced unexplainable **breathlessness at rest** (episodic pulmonary edema) that is **relieved in a supine position and exacerbated by standing**. She also complains of significant **weight loss** over the past year.
PE	VS: **mild fever**. PE: pallor and clubbing; on auscultation, **S1 delayed and decreased in intensity** and characteristic **low-pitched sound** (tumor plop) **during early diastole**, followed by a rumble; **auscultatory findings vary with body position**.
Labs	CBC: normochromic, normocytic anemia. **Elevated ESR**; increased IgG; blood cultures sterile. ECG: **sinus rhythm**.
Imaging	Echo (2D): characteristic echo-producing **mass in left atrium**. MR, cardiac: globular **mass** in left atrium.
Gross Pathology	Single globular left atrial mass about 6 cm in diameter, pedunculated with fibrovascular stalk arising from **interatrial septum** in vicinity of **fossa ovalis** (favored site of atrial origin).
Micro Pathology	**Stellate, multipotential mesenchymal myxoma cells** mixed with **endothelial cells**; mature and immature smooth muscle cells and macrophages, all in an **acid mucopolysaccharide matrix**.
Treatment	**Surgical excision** using cardiopulmonary bypass is curative.
Discussion	The **most common type of primary cardiac tumors**, myxomas may be located in any of the four chambers or, rarely, in the valves. They are **predominantly atrial with a 4:1 left-to-right ratio** and are **usually single**. Their signs and symptoms are closely related to their location and to the patient's position. Although myxomas are benign, they can embolize, resulting in metastatic disease. Although most myxomas are sporadic, some are familial with **autosomal-dominant** transmission; thus, echocardiographic **screening** of first-degree relatives is appropriate.
Atlas Link	[U][C][M][I] PG-P1-006

ID/CC	A **78-year-old** white **male** is brought into the emergency room with **nausea, dyspnea**, and a **crushing substernal chest pain** that **radiates** to his **left arm and jaw**; the pain has lasted for about 30 minutes and is not relieved with rest.
HPI	One sublingual nitroglycerin tablet did not relieve his pain. His history reveals a **sedentary lifestyle, moderate hypercholesterolemia**, and **obesity**. The patient is also a **diabetic** and **smokes**.
PE	VS: hypotension. PE: **diaphoresis**.
Labs	ECG: **ST elevation** with peaking of T waves; subsequent development of **inverted T waves** and **permanent Q waves**. Later, ST and T waves normalize. **Elevated CK-MB; elevated troponin T and I**. CBC: leukocytosis.
Imaging	Echo: **decreased wall motion** (HYPOKINESIS).
Gross Pathology	12 hours: no myocardial damage; 24 hours: pallor due to coagulation necrosis or reddish mottling; 3 to 5 days: demarcated yellow region with hyperemic border; 2 to 3 weeks: soft, gelatinous; 1 to 2 months: white scar and firm, thin wall.
Micro Pathology	12 to 18 hours: nuclear pyknosis, **coagulation necrosis**, and eosinophilia; 1 to 3 days: intense neutrophilic infiltrate, loss of nuclei and cross-striations; 1 week: disappearance of PMNs, onset of fibroblastic repair; 3 weeks: granulation tissue with progressive fibrosis.
Treatment	Oxygen, bed rest, aspirin, pain relief with morphine, nitrates, beta-blockers; plaque stabilization with heparin, anti-Gp IIa-IIIb monoclonal antibodies; thrombolysis with tPA if cardiac catheterization is not immediately available; cardiac catheterization with angioplasty or surgical reperfusion with a bypass graft depending on nature of disease; ACE inhibitors (limit postinfarct remodeling) and cholesterol-lowering drugs.
Discussion	The most common cause of myocardial infarction is atherosclerosis (coronary artery disease); it is less commonly caused by coronary vasospasm (Prinzmetal's angina). Sequelae include arrhythmias, congestive heart failure, pulmonary edema, shock, pulmonary embolism, papillary muscle rupture, ventricular aneurysm, ventricular wall rupture, tamponade, and autoimmune fibrinous pericarditis (DRESSLER'S SYNDROME).
Atlas Links	UCV1 PG-P1-007, PM-P1-007

CAD—MYOCARDIAL INFARCTION

ID/CC	A 50-year-old male who was admitted to the CCU **3 days ago** following an **MI** presents with **hypotension**.
HPI	The patient was thrombolyzed post-MI and was recovering well. He also complained of a mild fever but no chills or rigors.
PE	VS: tachycardia; weak, thready pulse; tachypnea; **hypotension**. PE: pallor; cool, moist skin; mild cyanosis of lips and digits; > 10-mmHg fall in arterial pressure with inspiration (PULSUS PARADOXUS); **heart sounds muffled** and **JVP elevated**; lungs clear bilaterally.
Labs	Elevated cardiac enzymes (CK-MB, troponin) as a result of recent acute MI.
Imaging	Echo: diastolic compression of the right ventricle; pericardial effusion.
Gross Pathology	Rupture of the left ventricular wall with hemopericardium.
Micro Pathology	Ischemic coagulative necrosis of the affected myocardium, consisting of multiple erythrocytes and dead, anucleated myocytes.
Treatment	Emergency pericardiocentesis; treat shock by infusing fluid and isoproterenol; surgical repair of cardiac rupture subsequent to stabilization.
Discussion	Cardiac rupture most typically develops 3 to 10 days after the initial onset of the infarction secondary to rupture of necrotic cardiac muscle; there is usually little warning before the sudden collapse, which is associated with acute cardiac tamponade and electromechanical dissociation. Papillary muscle rupture may also occur following an acute MI, resulting in mitral regurgitation and left ventricular failure.

ID/CC   A 60-year-old male presents to a clinic for a **heart transplant evaluation**.

HPI   The patient was diagnosed last year with **class III** (marked limitation of activity; comfortable only at rest) **congestive heart failure** secondary to **idiopathic dilated cardiomyopathy**. He is currently being treated with digoxin, furosemide (diuretic), lisinopril (ACE inhibitor), and warfarin (anticoagulant) but continues to be symptomatic.

PE   VS: normal. PE: elevated JVP; S3/S4 gallop heard on auscultation; significant pitting lower extremity **edema**.

Labs   CBC/Lytes: Normal. TFTs, LFTs, total protein, albumin, uric acid, and 24-hour protein/creatinine normal; PSA normal; IgG and IgM antibody titers against CMV, HSV, HIV, VZV, hepatitis B and C, and toxoplasmosis negative; PT/PTT/INR normal.

Imaging   Echo: EF 15% with moderate mitral valve regurgitation. CXR: **cardiomegaly**. ECG: occasional **premature ventricular contractions (PVCs)**. Thallium scan: **exercise-induced global cardiac ischemia**.

Treatment   If approved as a viable transplant candidate, the patient must wait for a suitable donor (matched according to body size, weight, **ABO blood grouping**, and levels of **panel reactive antibody**, or **PRA**). About 24% of patients waiting for a cardiac transplant (CT) die before a donor can be found. Most cardiac transplants are **orthotopic**.

Discussion   Cardiac transplantation accounts for 14% of organ transplant procedures and can dramatically improve cardiac function in individuals with end-stage cardiac disease. Patients must have **New York Heart Association (NYHA) class III or IV congestive heart failure**, having failed maximum medical therapy and other therapeutic interventions such as PCTA for CAD. Currently, **ischemic heart disease** accounts for approximately 55% of causes requiring CT and **idiopathic cardiomyopathy** for roughly 40%.

ID/CC	A 65-year-old white male complains of **requiring three pillows in bed in order to breathe comfortably** (ORTHOPNEA) and having to open the window to **gasp for air at night** (PAROXYSMAL NOCTURNAL DYSPNEA).
HPI	He has also noted **increasing shortness of breath** while walking as well as **swelling of his ankles and legs**. He had a **myocardial infarction** 2 years ago and has a history of **chronic hypertension**.
PE	VS: tachycardia; tachypnea; weak, thready pulse. PE: central cyanosis; **distention of neck veins** (due to elevated JVP); **third heart sound**; grade III/VI crescendo aortic systolic murmur; **crepitant rales** over both lower lobes; **lower lung fields dull to percussion** bilaterally; tender hepatomegaly; 4+ **pitting edema** in both lower extremities; cold extremities.
Labs	ABGs: hypoxemia; **low cardiac output** as measured by Fick equation and Swan-Ganz catheter (2.4 L/min); transudate in pleural fluid; increased BUN. ECG: left ventricular hypertrophy.
Imaging	CXR: enlarged cardiac silhouette; bilateral pleural effusions and diffuse increased lung markings (KERLEY B LINES) suggesting pulmonary edema. Echo: **ejection fraction of 40%**.
Gross Pathology	Cardiomegaly due to both dilatation and hypertrophy; pulmonary edema with increase in weight and reddish-purple color; nutmeg liver (due to chronic passive congestion).
Micro Pathology	Hepatization of lungs with alveolar capillary congestion and alveolar macrophages with hemosiderin ("HEART FAILURE CELLS"); centrilobular liver congestion.
Treatment	**Diuretics; low-sodium diet, digoxin; ACE inhibitors**; nitrates; antiarrhythmics.
Discussion	Congestive heart failure (CHF) is heart failure due to a deficit in myocardial strength or to an increase in workload. CHF is a common complication of ischemic and hypertensive heart disease in older populations.
Atlas Links	Ⓤ🅒🅜🆅🅘 PG-P1-010A, PG-P1-010B

ID/CC   A 35-year-old female **Asian** immigrant complains of weakness, **shortness of breath on exertion**, and **swelling of both feet**.

HPI   She also complains of **progressive abdominal distention** and fatigue. She was treated for **pulmonary tuberculosis** a few years ago.

PE   VS: mild hypotension; **reduced pulse pressure**. PE: peripheral cyanosis and cold extremities; pallor; neck veins distended; **JVP increases during inspiration** (KUSSMAUL'S SIGN); pedal edema; moderate hepatomegaly, splenomegaly, and ascites; **reduced-intensity apical impulse, distant heart sounds, and early third heart sound (pericardial knock)**; no pulsus paradoxus; no murmur or rub heard.

Labs   ECG: **low-voltage** QRS complexes with flattening of T wave (nonspecific). LFTs mildly abnormal (due to hepatic congestion); ascitic fluid **transudative** (low protein, high sugar). UA: proteinuria, no casts.

Imaging   CXR: **fibrosis** (old healed tuberculosis); heart shadow shows signs of **pericardial calcification**. Echo: **pericardial thickening**. CT: pericardial **calcification** and **thickening**.

Gross Pathology   Thick, dense, **fibrous obliteration of pericardial space with calcification** encasing the heart and **limiting diastolic filling**.

Treatment   **Complete pericardial resection** is the only definitive treatment; institute **antituberculous therapy** when appropriate; diuretics; sodium restriction; digitalis for associated atrial fibrillation (in one-third of patients).

Discussion   The etiology of constrictive pericarditis lies in the formation of scar tissue that encases the heart and interferes with ventricular filling. **Tuberculosis** is the most common cause worldwide. Most cases now seen in the United States are idiopathic, but cases resulting from exposure to **radiation**, trauma, cardiac surgery, rheumatoid arthritis, or uremia have become more common.

ID/CC	A 60-year-old white male who has been treated for **COPD** comes to the emergency room with severe **dyspnea at rest**.
HPI	Over the past few months, the patient has noted an **increased productive cough** and **exertional dyspnea**. He admits to being a **heavy smoker** and failed to quit smoking even after the appearance of **symptoms and the diagnosis of COPD**.
PE	**Elevated JVP** with large a and v waves; **loud P2**; cyanosis; clubbing of fingers; bilateral wheezing; expiratory rhonchi; prolonged expiration; use of accessory muscles of respiration; left parasternal heave; **ankle and sacral edema; tender hepatomegaly**.
Labs	ECG: **right-axis deviation** and **peaked P waves** (P PULMONALE). PFTs: COPD pattern.
Imaging	CXR: right ventricular and **pulmonary artery enlargement; hyperinflation**.
Gross Pathology	Right ventricular hypertrophy.
Treatment	Oxygen; salt and water restriction; treatment of COPD.
Discussion	Cor pulmonale is **right heart failure due to a pulmonary cause**, most commonly COPD. Other causes are pulmonary fibrosis, pneumoconioses, recurrent pulmonary embolism, primary pulmonary hypertension, obesity with sleep apnea, cystic fibrosis, bronchiectasis, and kyphoscoliosis.

ID/CC. A 29-year-old female who **recently gave birth** to a healthy infant develops **dyspnea** and **swelling of her feet** toward the end of the day.

HPI She is nursing her 6-week-old child.

PE VS: BP mildly elevated. PE: JVP raised with prominent a and v waves; tender, mild hepatosplenomegaly; cardiac apex heaving and displaced outside midclavicular line; **pansystolic apical murmur** (due to **mitral insufficiency**) and systolic murmur increasing with inspiration heard in tricuspid area (due to tricuspid insufficiency); loud pulmonary component of S2; S3 and S4 gallop; fine inspiratory basal crepitant rales at both lung bases; pedal edema.

Labs ECG: premature ventricular contractions.

Imaging CXR: interstitial pulmonary edema (due to severe pulmonary venous hypertension); **global cardiomegaly**. Echo/Nuc: cardiomegaly with diminished ventricular contractility (**systolic dysfunction**). Stress test: **decreased ejection fraction with stress** (ejection fraction normally increases with stress).

Gross Pathology Global dilatation of all chambers.

Micro Pathology **Extensive fibrosis without active inflammation** on endocardial biopsy.

Treatment Cardiac failure treated with salt restriction, diuretics, vasodilators, **ACE inhibitors**, and digoxin; chronic **anticoagulation**; nutritional supplementation; consider cardiac transplant if medical therapy fails.

Discussion Dilated cardiomyopathy usually develops in the **peripartum period** (± 3 months). Other etiologies include **alcoholism** (due to thiamine deficiency or direct toxicity), hypothyroidism, Friedreich's ataxia, previous **myocarditis** (usually due to **coxsackie B**), myotonic dystrophy, chronic hypocalcemia or hypophosphatemia, **sarcoidosis**, and drug toxicities (e.g., **adriamycin**, cyclophosphamide, **tricyclic antidepressants**, **lithium**, and cobalt).

Atlas Link ⬚⬚⬚⬚ PG-P1-013

ID/CC A 23-year-old woman is seen with complaints of **excessive breathlessness, palpitations, fatigue, blood-streaked sputum** (MILD HEMOPTYSIS), **and swelling of the feet** (EDEMA).

HPI She was diagnosed with **ventricular septal defect** (VSD) at birth, but her parents had refused surgery.

PE VS: HR, BP normal; mild tachypnea; no fever. PE: **central cyanosis**; clubbing; JVP normal; left parasternal heave; P2 palpable; single second heart sound, predominantly loud P2 (due to pulmonary hypertension); pansystolic murmur along left sternal edge; ejection systolic murmur in pulmonary area; **mid-diastolic murmur** (GRAHAM STEELL MURMUR OF PULMONARY REGURGITATION) **in pulmonary area that increased with inspiration** (CARVALLO'S SIGN, INDICATING RIGHT-SIDED MURMUR).

Labs ABGs: hypercapnia, hypoxia, and partly compensated respiratory acidosis. CBC: **polycythemia**. ECG: **right ventricular hypertrophy** with right-axis deviation. Cardiac catheterization reveals right-to-left shunt, **pulmonary arterial hypertension**, and pulmonary regurgitation.

Imaging Echo (with Doppler): **VSD with right-to-left systolic shunt**; right ventricular enlargement and hypertrophy. CXR: pulmonary oligemia ("peripheral pruning") and greatly enlarged hilar pulmonary artery shadows; cardiomegaly.

Treatment Heart-lung transplantation; surgical correction of a VSD is ideally performed before irreversible pulmonary vascular changes set in.

Discussion The term "Eisenmenger's syndrome" applies to those defects in which **pulmonary vascular disease causes right-to-left shunt of blood**; Eisenmenger's complex is right-to-left shunt due to a large VSD. The risk of infective endocarditis is high; therefore, antimicrobial prophylaxis is mandatory. Pregnancy is contraindicated owing to a high maternal mortality rate.

ID/CC A 20-year-old college student is brought back from a summer camp in the mountains after developing **severe shortness of breath** (DYSPNEA), cough with **blood-tinged sputum** (HEMOPTYSIS), and wheezing.

HPI The group had **ascended to a height** of **8,000 feet** and had engaged in **strenuous physical activities**. The patient subsequently developed dyspnea and cough that worsened during the night, leading to **marked respiratory distress and a shock-like state**.

PE VS: tachycardia; tachypnea; hypotension. PE: **central cyanosis**; pale and cold extremities; marked **respiratory distress; widespread rales and rhonchi** over both lung fields.

Labs CBC: **elevated hematocrit and hemoglobin**; mildly increased WBC. ABGs: markedly **decreased arterial PO_2** (hypoxia); **low PCO_2. Increased pH** (respiratory alkalosis). ECG: sinus tachycardia with **acute pulmonary hypertension**.

Imaging CXR (PA view): **noncardiogenic pulmonary edema** and prominent main pulmonary artery.

Micro Pathology Extensive pulmonary edema; protein-rich exudate with alveolar hemorrhages and **alveolar hyaline membranes**.

Treatment **Prompt descent, hyperbaric oxygen inhalation, sublingual nifedipine (after checking blood pressure)**, and placement in **portable hyperbaric chamber** while being transported; hospital management consists of **continuous high-flow oxygen, dexamethasone for CNS symptoms, and acetazolamide**.

Discussion High-altitude pulmonary edema is primarily a disorder of the pulmonary circulation **induced by sustained alveolar hypoxia**. The initiating event is an abnormal degree of **hypoxia-induced pulmonary arteriolar (precapillary) constriction** (hypoxia causes dilatation of systemic blood vessels) that elevates pulmonary arterial pressure. The imbalance of **increased blood flow** and pressure allows fluid to leave the pulmonary vasculature, resulting in **edema**.

ID/CC	A 21-year-old white male presents with anginal chest pain, **dyspnea on exertion**, and an episode of **syncope while playing basketball**.
HPI	The patient has no history of blue spells, squatting for relief, or rheumatic fever in childhood.
PE	VS: pulse bisferious (DOUBLE PEAKED). PE: JVP normal; cardiac apex forceful with strong presystolic impulse (DOUBLE APICAL IMPULSE); systolic thrill palpable over left sternal border; **S4; ejection systolic murmur** over left third intercostal space radiating to base and axilla; murmur **increased by exercise and during forced expiration against a closed glottis** (VALSALVA MANEUVER) but **decreased by squatting**.
Labs	ECG: left-axis deviation due to **left ventricular hypertrophy**; Q wave exaggerated in inferior and lateral precordial leads (due to septal hypertrophy).
Imaging	CXR, PA: often normal. Echo: **asymmetrical septal hypertrophy and systolic anterior motion of mitral valve**; Doppler may show **mitral regurgitation**. Angio, cardiac: marked **thickening of left ventricular septal wall**; small ventricular cavity with impaired ventricular filling (diastolic dysfunction) and narrow outflow tract ("HOURGLASS" APPEARANCE).
Gross Pathology	**Enlarged heart** with increased weight and **asymmetrical septal hypertrophy**.
Micro Pathology	Myocyte disarray with increased norepinephrine content.
Treatment	Negative inotropic agents (e.g., **beta-blockers**) to decrease stiffness of left ventricle and prevent fatal arrhythmias; **avoidance of competitive sports**; amiodarone (may be useful in prevention of lethal cardiac arrhythmias); surgical myomectomy of interventricular septum in patients with outflow obstruction.
Discussion	Also known as **idiopathic hypertrophic subaortic stenosis (IHSS)**. An **autosomal-dominant** pattern of disease is noted in 50% of cases; ventricular outflow tract obstruction by hypertrophy produces symptoms. The presenting symptom in **athletes** might be **sudden death** secondary to lethal cardiac arrhythmias.
Atlas Link	UCV1 PG-P1-016

HYPERTROPHIC OBSTRUCTIVE CARDIOMYOPATHY

ID/CC A 28-year-old woman **found on a park bench apparently dead** is brought to the ER in the early hours of the morning.

HPI No discernible pulse was palpated, but a **faint, infrequent respiratory effort was noted**; CPR was begun and continued during her transport to the hospital. The **temperature overnight was near-freezing** with continuous rain.

PE VS: arterial **pulse not palpated**; hypotension; reduced respiratory rate; **severe hypothermia (< 28°C)**. PE: no respiratory effort; **fixed and dilated pupils**; blotchy areas of erythema on skin; bullae over buttocks; chest exam shows diffuse rales bilaterally; absent bowel sounds; absent deep tendon reflexes.

Labs CBC: increased hematocrit. Hypoglycemia; increased BUN and creatinine. Lytes: decreased bicarbonate; hyperkalemia. ABGs: severe metabolic acidosis. ECG: evidence of **marked bradycardia with J (Osborn) waves** (upward waves immediately following the S wave).

Imaging CXR: patchy atelectasis.

Treatment Intubation and ventilation as necessary; cardiac massage for arrest; warm the patient through use of a combination of heated blankets, heat packs, warm gastric lavage, warm-water immersion, and high-flow oxygen; monitor cardiac rhythm for arrhythmias.

Discussion Hypothermia is defined as core temperature below 35°C; **severe accidental hypothermia (below 30°C, or 86°F) is associated with marked depression in cerebral blood flow and cerebral oxygen requirement, reduced cardiac output, and decreased arterial pressure**. Victims can **appear to be lifeless** as a result of marked depression of brain function. Peripheral pulses may be difficult to detect because of bradycardia and vasoconstriction. Complications of systemic hypothermia may include ventricular fibrillation, pancreatitis, renal failure, and coagulopathy.

ID/CC	A 42-year-old black male presents with **chest pain, headache, altered mental status, and confusion**.
HPI	He is known to have **labile essential hypertension**. He has no history of fever.
PE	VS: **severe diastolic hypertension** (BP 230/150). PE: **disoriented and confused; bilateral papilledema**; no focal neurologic deficits; remainder of exam normal.
Labs	CBC: microangiopathic hemolytic anemia. UA: **hematuria** and **proteinuria. Increased BUN and serum creatinine. ECG: left ventricular hypertrophy**.
Imaging	CT/US, abdomen: bilateral **small and scarred kidneys**.
Gross Pathology	Kidney surface appears **"flea-bitten"** (due to rupture of cortical arterioles and glomerular capillaries).
Micro Pathology	Renal biopsy (not routinely indicated) shows **hyperplastic arteriolosclerosis** ("ONION SKINNING") of interlobular arteries with **fibrinoid necrosis** and thrombi in arterioles and small arteries; **necrotizing glomerulitis** with neutrophil infiltration also seen.
Treatment	IV **sodium nitroprusside** or IV beta-blockers in conjunction with 24-hour cardiac monitoring in acute phase; subsequent management with oral antihypertensives and emphasis on strict patient compliance.
Discussion	**End-organ damage** caused by malignant hypertension includes hemorrhagic and lacunar strokes, encephalopathy, fundal hemorrhages, papilledema, myocardial ischemia/infarction, left ventricular hypertrophy, congestive heart failure, acute renal failure, nephrosclerosis, aortic dissection, and necrotizing vasculitis.
Atlas Links	**UCV1** PG-P1-018, PM-P1-018 **UCV2** ER-005

ID/CC   The case of a 50-year-old man who died of bleeding complications is discussed at an autopsy meeting owing to **peculiar vegetations seen on his mitral valve**.

HPI   He underwent surgery for **adenocarcinoma of the stomach**. Shortly before his death he was diagnosed as having **disseminated intravascular coagulation (DIC)**; he subsequently died of bleeding complications.

Gross Pathology   **Small** (1- to 5-mm) **friable, sterile vegetations** loosely adherent to **mitral valve leaflets along lines of closure**.

Micro Pathology   Vegetations found to be **sterile fibrin and platelet thrombi** loosely attached **without evidence of inflammation** (bland) or valve damage.

Discussion   Nonbacterial thrombotic endocarditis characteristically occurs in settings of **prolonged debilitating diseases** such as cancer (particularly visceral adenocarcinomas), DIC, renal failure, chronic sepsis, or other **hypercoagulable states**. The vegetations may produce emboli and subsequent infarctions in the heart, kidneys, brain, mesentery, or extremities.

ID/CC	A 37-year-old white male complains of increasing **fatigue** and shortness of breath **during minimal physical exertion**.
HPI	He denies having had any chest pain or having any previous history of similar symptoms. A careful history reveals **rheumatic fever** at age 7.
PE	VS: jerky pulse (RAPID UPSTROKE). PE: high-pitched **pansystolic murmur** at **apex with radiation to axilla**; S3.
Labs	ECG: left-axis deviation; left atrial and left ventricular hypertrophy.
Imaging	CXR/Echo: enlargement of left atrium and ventricle. Doppler: confirmatory.
Treatment	Oral arteriolar vasodilators (e.g., ACE inhibitors, hydralazine) to improve forward cardiac output; surgical repair or prosthetic replacement; antibiotic prophylaxis with penicillin prior to surgical or dental procedures.
Discussion	Common causes of mitral insufficiency include **mitral valve prolapse**, ischemic papillary muscle dysfunction, infective endocarditis, hypertrophic cardiomyopathy, ventricular enlargement, mitral annulus calcification, and dilated cardiomyopathy; rheumatic heart disease is no longer the leading cause.

ID/CC A 34-year-old white female in her 27th week of pregnancy is admitted to the hospital with **dyspnea** and **orthopnea**.

HPI The patient denies any prior cardiovascular disease, but a careful history reveals that she suffered from **streptococcal pharyngitis** and **rheumatic heart disease** as a child.

PE Malar flush; elevated JVP (due to venous congestion); left parasternal heave; loud S1; **opening snap**; rumbling, low-pitched **mid-diastolic murmur** at **apex** heard best in left lateral position.

Labs ECG: **left atrial hypertrophy** and/or **atrial fibrillation**.

Imaging CXR: double silhouette due to enlarged left atrium; Kerley B lines (due to interstitial edema). Echo: **leaflet thickening** with **fusion of the commissures**.

Gross Pathology Thickened and scarred mitral valve.

Treatment Treat atrial fibrillation; anticoagulation, commissurotomy, prosthetic valve replacement; antibiotic prophylaxis prior to surgical or dental procedures; diuretics to relieve pulmonary congestion.

Discussion The most common cause of mitral stenosis is rheumatic heart disease. The main changes to the valve include leaflet thickening, fusion of the commissures, and shortening, thickening, and fusion of the cordae tendineae.

ID/CC	An 18-year-old white **male** complains of gradually progressing **shortness of breath** and **ankle swelling**.
HPI	His symptoms started following a **URI**. He also complains of **excessive fatigue and frequent chest pain**. He has no history of joint pain, skin rash, or involuntary movements (vs. rheumatic fever) and is neither hypertensive nor diabetic.
PE	VS: tachycardia; hypotension; no fever. PE: **elevated JVP**; pitting pedal edema; fine inspiratory rales at both lung bases; mild tender hepatomegaly; splenomegaly; **right-sided S3**; murmurs of mitral regurgitation.
Labs	ASO titers not raised. CBC: lymphocytosis. Elevated ESR. ECG: **first-degree AV block with nonspecific ST-T** changes. **Coxsackievirus** isolated on pharyngeal washings; increased titers of serum antibodies to coxsackievirus; **elevated cardiac enzymes**.
Imaging	CXR: cardiomegaly and pulmonary edema. Echo: suggestive of dilated cardiomyopathy with low ejection fraction.
Gross Pathology	Flabby, dilated heart with foci of myocardial petechial hemorrhages.
Micro Pathology	Endomyocardial biopsy reveals **diffuse infiltration by mononuclear cells, predominantly lymphocytes**; interstitial edema; focal myofiber necrosis; focal fibrosis.
Treatment	Rest; specific antimicrobial therapy when appropriate; control of congestive cardiac failure by diuretics, digitalis, and vasodilators; antiarrhythmics if indicated; cardiac transplant in intractable cases. Although most cases of acute myocarditis may resolve spontaneously, some progress to dilated cardiomyopathy.
Discussion	The etiology of myocarditis is usually **coxsackie B** or other viruses; less often implicated are bacteria or fungi, rickettsiae (e.g., Rocky Mountain spotted fever), spirochetes (e.g., Lyme disease), *Trypanosoma cruzi* (Chagas' disease), hypersensitivity disease (SLE, drug reaction), radiation, and sarcoidosis. Diphtheria toxin also causes myocarditis by inhibiting eukaryotic elongation factor 2 (EF-2), thus inhibiting myocyte protein synthesis. It may also be idiopathic. Young males are primarily affected.

ID/CC   A 64-year-old white female complains of **sudden-onset severe pain** in her left leg with **associated weakness** of the left foot. The pain intensifies when she moves her leg, and she cannot move her toes at all.

HPI   She is a **smoker** and has a history of **limited exercise tolerance** due to **pain in her lower extremities** (INTERMITTENT CLAUDICATION).

PE   VS: normal. PE: lipid deposition in skin (XANTHELASMAS); popliteal, dorsalis pedis, and posterior tibial **pulses lost** on left side; femoral pulses easily palpable; left leg **cold and mottled; anesthesia** over lower left leg.

Labs   CBC: leukocytosis.

Imaging   US, Doppler: obstruction of left femoral artery at origin. Angio: confirmatory; assess runoff and collaterals prior to surgery.

Treatment   Thrombolysis; consider embolectomy.

Discussion   Arterial embolism may have various causes, such as **atrial fibrillation, myocardial infarction, prosthetic heart valves**, endocarditis, cancer, dilated cardiomyopathy, **paradoxical embolism** from the venous system, or a dislodged mural thrombus from an **abdominal aortic aneurysm** or an atheromatous plaque. The earlier the intervention, the higher the likelihood that the limb may be salvaged. Clinically characterized by the **five P's: pain, pallor, paralysis, paresthesia, and pulselessness.**

ID/CC A 25-year-old male is brought to the ER after having sustained a stab wound on his left thigh following a drunken brawl.

HPI A tourniquet was tied above the site, which the attendants said was **spurting blood like "a tap run open."**

PE VS: **hypotension**; weak, fast pulse. PE: anxious and confused; **cool skin with reduced capillary filling**; very **low central venous pressure**; releasing tourniquet confirmed femoral artery puncture.

Labs CBC: mildly decreased hematocrit. BUN and creatinine normal. Lytes: normal.

Imaging Arteriogram shows abrupt termination of dye propagation in the common femoral artery.

Treatment Arrest of femoral artery hemorrhage with vascular repair; intensive IV fluid therapy using normal saline and cross-matched blood transfusions; supplemental oxygen; close monitoring of pulse rate, blood pressure, urine output, and central venous pressure.

Discussion The clinical conditions that cause hypovolemic shock include **acute and subacute hemorrhage and dehydration**; fluid loss into an extravascular compartment can significantly reduce intravascular volume and result in nonhemorrhagic hypovolemic shock. Acute pancreatitis, loss of the enteral integument (from conditions such as burns and surgical wounds), or occlusive or dynamic ileus can all induce oligemic hypotension as a result of extravasation of fluids into the extracellular compartment. Other forms of water and solute loss, such as diarrhea, hyperglycemia (leading to glucosuria), diabetes insipidus, salt-wasting nephritis, protracted vomiting, adrenocortical failure, acute peritonitis, and overzealous use of diuretics, can also lead to decreased intravascular volume and hypovolemic shock. Patients with prolonged tissue hypoperfusion may progress to metabolic acidosis.

ID/CC   A 29-year-old-male is referred to a cardiology clinic for evaluation for a permanent pacemaker.

HPI   The patient is asymptomatic and denies dizziness, syncope, chest pain, or shortness of breath. He was incidentally noted to have **sinus bradycardia**. He is a **marathon runner** and works as a ranger in a national park, often at elevations above 8,000 feet.

PE   VS: no fever, **mild hypotension (BP 90/50) without orthostasis; bradycardia (HR 40)**. PE: thin and athletic-looking; normal JVP; S1 and S2 normally auscultated without any murmurs, gallops, and/or rubs; no lower extremity edema.

Labs   CBC/Lytes: normal. ECG: marked **sinus bradycardia** with a ventricular rate of **40 beats/minute**.

Imaging   XR, chest: normal.

Treatment   In emergent situations, treat **symptomatic sinus bradycardia** with IV access, supplemental oxygen, and cardiac monitoring. IV atropine may be used in symptomatic patients. Correct all underlying electrolyte and acid-base disorders or hypoxia. Address cause of bradycardia. This patient has a **physiologic sinus bradycardia**, and thus no treatment is indicated.

Discussion   **Sinus bradycardia** is defined as a sinus rhythm with a resting heart rate of less than **60 beats/minute**. Physiologic causes of sinus bradycardia include **increased vagal tone** seen in athletes and incidental findings in **young** or **sleeping** patients. Pathologic causes include **inferior wall myocardial infarction, toxic or environmental exposure (dimethyl sulfoxide, toluene), electrolyte disorders, infection, sleep apnea, drug effects (digitalis glycosides, beta-blockers, amiodarone, calcium channel blockers), hypoglycemia, hypothyroidism**, and **increased intracranial pressure**. The most common cause of symptomatic sinus bradycardia is **sick sinus syndrome**.

ID/CC	A **35-year-old man** complains of severe, **cramping pains in his calves that prevent him from walking** (INTERMITTENT CLAUDICATION).
HPI	The patient states that the pain comes mainly after playing basketball. More recently it has appeared, accompanied by numbness, following mild exertion and **at rest** (due to progression of disease). He admits to **smoking** up to three packs of cigarettes per day.
PE	Painful, cordlike indurations of veins (sequelae of **migratory superficial thrombophlebitis**); **pallor**; cyanosis; coldness; diminished peripheral artery pulsations; **Raynaud's phenomenon**; delayed return of hand color following release of temporarily occluded radial artery while exercising hand.
Imaging	Angio, peripheral: **multiple occluded segments** of small and medium-sized arteries in lower leg.
Gross Pathology	Arterial segmental thrombosis; **no atherosclerosis**; secondary **gangrene** of leg if severe.
Micro Pathology	Segmental vasculitis with round cell infiltration in **all layers** of arterial wall; inflammation; thrombosis; microabscess formation.
Treatment	**Cessation of smoking** critical; sympathectomy; amputation.
Discussion	Thromboangiitis obliterans tends to affect medium-size and small arteries of the distal extremities. If smoking is not discontinued, multiple finger and toe amputations may be necessary.

THROMBOANGIITIS OBLITERANS (BUERGER'S DISEASE)

ID/CC	A 50-year-old female who was admitted to the hospital for treatment of staphylococcal endocarditis complains of **severe pain at the site of antibiotic infusion**.
HPI	She was receiving **cloxacillin** (has propensity to cause thrombophlebitis) in addition to penicillin and gentamycin.
PE	Markedly **tender, cordlike inflamed area** found at site of infusion.
Gross Pathology	Intraluminal venous thrombus adherent to the vessel wall.
Micro Pathology	Acute inflammatory cells with endothelial wall damage and intraluminal thrombosis.
Treatment	Change infusion site frequently; NSAIDs and local heat; support and bed rest.
Discussion	Superficial thrombophlebitis most commonly occurs in **varicose veins** or in **veins cannulated for an infusion**. Spontaneous thrombophlebitis may occur in conditions such as pregnancy, polycythemia, polyarteritis nodosa, and Buerger's disease (thromboangiitis obliterans) and as a sign of visceral cancer (thrombophlebitis migrans—Trousseau's sign).

ID/CC A 15-year-old boy is referred to a cardiologist by a primary care physician for an evaluation of **recurrent dizzy spells**.

HPI During his episodes he feels **intense anxiety with palpitations and breathlessness**. He has no history of chest pain or syncope and is normal in between episodes of dizziness.

PE General and systemic physical exam normal; cardiac exam normal; otologic causes ruled out.

Labs ECG: **short PR interval, wide QRS complex, and a slurred upstroke** ("DELTA WAVE") **of QRS complex; R wave in V1 positive**. Electrophysiologic studies confirm **presence of a bypass tract** and its potential for development of life-threatening arrhythmia.

Treatment **Catheter radiofrequency ablation** of the accessory tract is the treatment of choice. Since digitalis reduces the refractory period of the accessory tract, it should be avoided.

Discussion Wolff–Parkinson–White (WPW) syndrome is a term that is applied to patients with both preexcitation on ECG and paroxysmal tachycardia; in this case, the spells of dizziness could have been either paroxysmal supraventricular tachycardia or atrial fibrillation. In WPW syndrome, an accessory pathway (Kent's bundle) exists between the atria and ventricles. An atrial premature contraction or a ventricular premature contraction generally initiates the reentrant tachycardia, with the accessory tract usually conducting in a retrograde manner; the danger of atrial fibrillation lies in the fact that the accessory pathway may be capable of conducting very fast atrial rates, leading to a fast ventricular response that may degenerate into ventricular arrhythmias.

ID/CC	A **60-year-old white** male **farmer** presents with skin lesions on his **forehead, above his upper lip, and on the dorsum of his hands**.
HPI	He does not smoke, drink alcohol, or chew tobacco.
PE	Round or irregularly shaped lesions; tan plaques with adherent **scaly or rough surface** on forehead, skin over upper lip, forearms, and dorsum of hands; lesions range in size from several millimeters to 1 cm or more.
Micro Pathology	Epidermis thickened with basal cell hyperplasia; atypical cells tend to invade most superficial portion of the dermis, which shows thickening and fibrosis (ELASTOSIS).
Treatment	Liquid-nitrogen cryotherapy; topical treatment with fluorouracil; surgical excision; electrodesiccation; minimize sun exposure.
Discussion	Also known as senile or **solar keratosis**, actinic keratosis is the most common **precancerous dermatosis** and may progress to **squamous cell carcinoma**. It occurs most commonly in **fair-skinned** individuals and in older persons. Signs that actinic keratosis has become malignant are elevation, ulceration or inflammation, and recent enlargement (> 1 cm). Immunosuppressed patients are at high risk of developing actinic keratosis with **prolonged sun exposure**. Look for multiple lesions and for newly developed lesions; **biopsy all suspicious lesions**.

ID/CC	A 12-year-old male presents with severe **itching** and burning at the back of both knees.
HPI	He has had similar episodes since the age of 7. His **mother** suffers from **asthma** and his **father** had a **similar skin ailment**.
PE	VS: no fever. PE: perioral pallor, increased palmar markings, and **extra fold of skin below the lower eyelid** (DENNIE'S LINE); **erythematous, vesicular, weeping, rough patchy skin rash** in both popliteal fossae with thickening, crusting, and scaling on the peripheries.
Labs	CBC: eosinophilia. High serum IgE levels.
Micro Pathology	Skin biopsy reveals lymphocytic infiltrate with edematous intercellular spaces in the epidermis and prominent intercellular bridges; splayed keratinocytes located primarily in the stratum spinosum.
Treatment	Avoidance of skin irritants; low- or midpotency **topical glucocorticoids**; antihistamines; systemic antibiotics (for secondary infection). Severe exacerbations unresponsive to topical steroids may need sysytemic steroids or immunosuppressive therapy.
Discussion	Clinical criteria for the diagnosis of atopic dermatitis include recurrent episodes of pruritus lasting more than 6 weeks with a personal or family history of atopy and skin lesions typical of eczematous dermatitis.

ID/CC	A 68-year-old **red-haired white** male presents with a 3-month history of a progressively **raised, bleeding, ulcerated lesion** over his upper lip that has not responded to various ointments.
HPI	He is a **farmer** and has always **worked outdoors**; he occasionally smokes but does not drink.
PE	Large, **ill-defined, telangiectatic and ulcerated nodule** ("PEARLY PAPULE") with heaped-up borders located over right upper lip; no regional lymphadenopathy.
Gross Pathology	Generally local but sometimes extensive destruction.
Micro Pathology	Biopsy shows basophilic cells with scant cytoplasm as well as palisading basal cells with atypia and increased mitotic index.
Treatment	Surgical excision with biopsy; cryosurgery; electrodesiccation.
Discussion	Basal cell carcinoma typically occurs in **light-skinned people**. **The most common skin cancer**, it is seen mainly on **sun-exposed areas** (e.g., face, nose) and is very slow-growing. **Metastatic disease is rare** ($< 0.17\%$); **chronic, prolonged exposure to sun** is the most important risk factor. Other risk factors include **male gender, advanced age, fair complexion**, and **outdoor occupations**. An increased incidence is seen in people with defective DNA repair mechanisms (e.g., xeroderma pigmentosum) and immunosuppression.
Atlas Links	UCV2 MC-335A, MC-335B

BASAL CELL CARCINOMA

ID/CC	An 8-year-old boy presents with **intense pruritus and fluid-filled blisters** over his arms and legs.
HPI	He recently went on a camping trip with his classmates, during which he played the whole day in the bushes around the camping site.
PE	Typical **linear streaked vesicles over both arms and legs**; weepy and encrusted areas; numerous scratch marks over skin.
Labs	Gram stain and culture to rule out secondary infection; KOH preparation negative.
Gross Pathology	Skin erythema and edema, with linear streaked vesicles.
Micro Pathology	Superficial perivascular **lymphocytic infiltration** around the blood vessels associated with edema of the dermal papillae and mast cell degranulation.
Treatment	Systemic and oral steroids.
Discussion	While at the campground the boy probably encountered poison ivy, a plant that produces low-molecular-weight oils (URUSHIOLS) that induce contact hypersensitivity, which is a **cell-mediated, type IV hypersensitivity reaction**. The antigen is presented by the Langerhans cells to the helper lymphocytes. Both cell types travel to regional lymph nodes, where the antigen presentation is increased. Upon antigen challenge, the sensitized T-cells infiltrate the dermis and begin the immune response.

ID/CC A 35-year-old **man** presents with an **intensely pruritic rash** on his **elbows, knees, and back.**

HPI He has **celiac sprue** and observes prescribed dietary precautions (gluten restriction).

PE PE: **bilaterally symmetrical** polymorphic skin lesions in the form of **small, tense vesicles on erythematous skin** (often in herpetiform groups); bullae and groups of papules over scapular and sacral areas, knees and elbows, and other **extensor surfaces.**

Labs **HLA-B8/DR-w3** haplotype (particularly prone).

Gross Pathology **Polymorphous erythematous lesions**, including **papules, small vesicles,** and **larger bullae.**

Micro Pathology Skin biopsy reveals characteristic **subepidermal blisters**, necrosis, and dermal papillary microabscesses; direct immunofluorescence studies reveal **granular deposits of IgA at tips of dermal papillae.**

Treatment **Dapsone therapy** after confirming adequate glucose-6-phosphate dehydrogenase (G6PD) levels (dapsone produces hemolysis in G6PD-deficient individuals).

Discussion Dermatitis herpetiformis is a vesicular and extremely pruritic skin disease **associated with gluten sensitivity enteropathy** and IgA immune complexes deposited in dermal papillae; individuals with HLA-B8/DR-w3 haplotype are predisposed to developing the disease. **Males** are often more commonly affected, and peak incidence is in the third and fourth decades. Patients on long-term dapsone therapy should be monitored for hemolysis and methemoglobinemia.

Atlas Link UCV2 IM2-005

ID/CC	A **16-year-old female** complains of **multiple nevi** on her skin.
HPI	She is concerned because an **aunt** who had a **similar illness** developed **malignant melanoma** and died of metastatic complications.
PE	**Multiple nevi measuring 6 to 15 mm** noted; nevi are variegated shades of pink, tan, and brown and seen on back, chest, buttocks, scalp, and breasts; **borders are irregular** and **poorly defined** but lack the scalloping of malignant melanoma; no regional lymphadenopathy noted.
Micro Pathology	Skin biopsy reveals melanocytes with **cytologic and architectural atypia**, enlarged and fused epidermal nevus cell nests, **lentiginous hyperplasia**, and **pigment incontinence**.
Treatment	Sun protection; regular skin exam to detect development of malignant melanoma and to biopsy suspicious lesions. Family members should be regularly monitored.
Discussion	Dysplastic nevi are found in individuals with an autosomal-dominant predisposition to develop acquired nevi; these **may develop into malignant melanoma.**
Atlas Link	UCV2 MC-135

ID/CC A 24-year-old female presents with a sudden-onset **skin rash** on both **forearms**.

HPI She suffers from **herpes labialis** and had a recent recurrence. Currently she is not taking any medications.

PE VS: normal. PE: **papulovesicular, erythematous skin lesions on both forearms**, occurring in **concentric rings with a clear center** (TARGET LESIONS); mucous membranes spared (vs. Stevens–Johnson syndrome).

Micro Pathology Skin biopsy reveals dermal edema and lymphocytic infiltrates intimately associated with degenerating keratinocytes along the dermal-epidermal junction; target lesions reveal a central necrosed area with a rim of perivenular inflammation.

Treatment **Treat underlying cause**, supportive therapy; **steroids** in severe cases.

Discussion Erythema multiforme is a hypersensitivity response to certain **drugs** (commonly sulfonamides, NSAIDs, penicillin, phenytoin) and **infections** (*Mycoplasma*, HSV). It is clinically divided into major and minor types. The minor type involves limited cutaneous surfaces, while the major type (STEVENS–JOHNSON SYNDROME) is characterized by toxic features and involvement of mucosal surfaces.

Atlas Link UCV2 MC-018

ID/CC A 24-year-old male presents with acute-onset, **painful swelling** in his **left axillae**.

HPI He also reports fever and a history of poorly controlled juvenile-onset diabetes mellitus.

PE VS: fever (39°C); tachycardia (HR 110). PE: multiple, mobile, **extremely tender, erythematous and fluctuant** axillary swellings; aspiration of swellings yields frank pus.

Labs CBC: **leukocytosis**. Gram stain of pus reveals gram-positive cocci in clusters; culture grows coagulase-positive *Staphylococcus aureus*.

Treatment **Incision and drainage**; systemic antibiotics (empiric penicillinase-resistant β-lactams; then according to reported culture sensitivities).

Discussion A boil (FURUNCLE) is a deep-seated infection of the hair follicle and adjacent subcutaneous tissue, most commonly occurring in moist hair bearing parts of the body. **Diabetes, HIV**, and **IV drug abuse** are predisposing conditions. Recurrent cutaneous infections with *S. aureus* may occur due to a chronic carrier state (most commonly in the anterior nares).

ID/CC	A 23-year-old **HIV-positive** man presents with **nonpruritic reddish-brown lesions**.
HPI	He has had a continuous low-grade fever, significant weight loss over the past 6 months, and painless lumps in the cervical, axillary, and inguinal areas.
PE	VS: fever. PE: emaciation; pallor; generalized lymphadenopathy; no hepatosplenomegaly or sternal tenderness; **reddish-purple plaques and nodules** over trunk and lower extremities; similar lesions noted in oral mucosa.
Labs	ELISA/Western blot positive for HIV. CBC/PBS: **lymphocytopenia with depressed CD4+ cell count** (< 100).
Gross Pathology	**Reddish-purple, raised plaques** and **firm nodules** with no suppuration.
Micro Pathology	Skin biopsy of nodular lesion shows malignant spindle cells with slitlike spaces containing RBCs, inflammatory cells, and hemosiderin-laden macrophages.
Treatment	Radiation; chemotherapy with etoposide or doxorubicin, bleomycin, α-interferon, and vinblastine. If iatrogenic, stop immunosuppressive medication.
Discussion	Kaposi's sarcoma is the **most common cancer associated with AIDS** (epidemic type). The non-AIDS type affects Ashkenazi Jews (chronic or classic type) and Africans (lymphadenopathic or endemic type), but the disease is not as aggressive. **Human herpesvirus 8** is associated with all types; **disordered cytokine regulation** also plays a role. Other than the skin, lesions are most commonly found in the **lymph nodes, GI tract**, and **lung**. In contrast to lymphoma, lymphadenopathy presents early and is not significant.
Atlas Link	UCV2 IM2-007

DERMATOLOGY

ID/CC	A 4-year-old Japanese male presents with **fever** and an **extensive skin rash**.
HPI	A primary care physician had previously found the patient to have cervical adenitis; antibiotics were administered but achieved no response.
PE	VS: fever. PE: **conjunctival congestion**; dry, red lips; **erythematous palms and soles**; indurative edema of peripheral extremities; **desquamation of fingertips**; various rashes of trunk; **cervical lymphadenopathy** > 1.5 cm.
Labs	**Throat swab and culture sterile**. CBC: routine blood counts normal; further differential blood counts reveal increased B-cell activation and T-helper-cell lymphocytopenia. Paul-Bunnell test for infectious mononucleosis negative; serologic tests rule out cytomegalovirus infection and toxoplasmosis.
Imaging	Angio: presence of **coronary artery aneurysms**.
Gross Pathology	Aneurysmal dilatation of the coronary arteries.
Micro Pathology	Coronary arteritis is usually demonstrated at autopsy together with aneurysm formation and thrombosis.
Treatment	Aspirin and IV gamma globulin are effective in preventing coronary complications if initiated early.
Discussion	Kawasaki's syndrome is usually self-limited, but in a few instances fatal coronary thrombosis has occurred during the acute stage of the disease or many months after apparently complete recovery. Case fatality rates have been about 1% to 2%.
Atlas Link	UCV2 MC-300

ID/CC　A 30-year-old **woman** is seen with an **itchy rash** over her **wrists, forearms**, and **trunk**.

HPI　She complains that fresh **lesions occur along scratch marks and areas of trauma** (KOEBNER'S PHENOMENON).

PE　VS: no fever. PE: polygonal, **purple, flat-topped papules and plaques; tiny white dots and lines over papules** (WICKHAM'S STRIAE); white netlike pattern of **lesions over oral mucosa**.

Gross Pathology　**Flat-topped, violaceous papules** and plaques **without scales**.

Micro Pathology　Dense, **bandlike (lichenoid) lymphocytic infiltrate** (predominantly T cells) along the dermal-epidermal junction; **sawtooth pattern of rete ridges**; destruction of basal cells.

Treatment　**Steroids**, topical (potent fluorinated) or systemic; **isotretinoin** is an effective alternative, but risk of **teratogenicity** must be borne in mind when prescribing.

Discussion　Lichen planus is a **self-limited inflammatory skin** disease, but in some cases it may be present for several years. Females are affected more frequently than males. Postinflammatory hyperpigmentation may be evident after the lesions subside. Medications such as tetracycline, penicillamine, and hydrochlorothiazide can cause lichen planus–like skin reactions.

Atlas Link　　UCV2　MC-142

ID/CC	A 50-year-old **white** male presents with an itchy, **rapidly enlarging, pigmented lesion** on the sole of his left foot.
HPI	He states that the spot has **recently changed color** dramatically; once lightly pigmented, it is now a deep purple hue.
PE	**Irregular, asymmetric, deeply pigmented lesion with various shades** of red and blue; diameter **> 6 mm**; left-sided nontender **inguinal lymphadenopathy**.
Gross Pathology	**Slightly raised**; deeply pigmented with uneven hues and irregular border.
Micro Pathology	Excisional biopsy shows tumor-free borders along with large, atypical, variably pigmented cells with irregular nuclei and eosinophilic nucleoli in epidermis and papillary dermis; dermal invasion noted in some places; metastases shown on lymph node biopsy.
Treatment	Excision with wide margin, regional lymph node dissection, chemotherapy, immunotherapy.
Discussion	Of all skin cancers, melanoma is responsible for the largest number of deaths. An increased incidence is seen in **fair-skinned** people and in those with **dysplastic nevi, immunosuppression**, and **excessive sun exposure**. Melanomas undergo a **radial (superficial) growth** phase followed by an invasive, **vertical growth** phase. **Bleeding, ulceration**, and **pain are late manifestations**. The **chance of metastasis increases with depth of invasion** (measured using Clark levels I–V). Metastatic melanomas are **incurable** and signify the **need for early detection** and prevention (e.g., sunblock, clothing).
Atlas Link	UCV2 SUR-004

MALIGNANT MELANOMA

ID/CC   A 60-year-old male presents with multiple lumps and a **chronic**, pruritic, erythematous **rash** that has spread and now **involves almost his entire body**.

HPI   He has seen many doctors, but the rash **has not responded to** a variety of medications, including **topical and systemic steroids**.

PE   Erythematous, circinate rash in **plaques** with **exfoliation** (SCALING); some **nodules** seen on face, trunk, lower abdomen, and buttocks; no regional lymphadenopathy or hepatosplenomegaly.

Labs   CBC/PBS: lymphocytosis.

Imaging   CXR: no mediastinal lymphadenopathy.

Gross Pathology   Reddish-brown, **kidney-shaped plaques** (vs. Hodgkin's lymphoma); hence name **"red man's disease"**; exfoliation, nodule formation, and sometimes ulceration.

Micro Pathology   Atypical, **PAS-positive, large, CD4-antigen-positive** (helper T-cell) **lymphocytes with characteristic multiconvoluted, "cerebriform" nuclei** (SÉZARY–LUTZNER CELLS); dermal infiltration with exocytosis of atypical mononuclear cells within epidermis found singly or within punched-out **epidermal microabscesses** (PAUTRIER'S ABSCESSES).

Treatment   PUVA; total skin electron-beam therapy; prednisone and chlorambucil or low-dose methotrexate.

Discussion   Mycosis fungoides is a malignant cutaneous helper T-cell lymphoma; disseminated disease with exfoliative dermatitis and generalized lymphadenopathy is termed **Sézary syndrome**.

Atlas Link   ⓤ🄲Ⓥ2 MC-144

ID/CC	A 25-year-old male is admitted to the hospital for an evaluation of **recurrent epistaxis**.
HPI	The patient's mother died of a **massive pulmonary hemorrhage due to an arteriovenous malformation**.
PE	**Small telangiectatic lesions** seen on lips, oral and nasal mucosa, tongue, and tips of fingers and toes; anemia noted; no pulmonary bruit heard (to detect an AV malformation).
Labs	CBC: normocytic, normochromic anemia (due to occult gastrointestinal blood loss). Guaiac positive.
Imaging	CT: AV malformations in liver and spleen.
Micro Pathology	Irregularly dilated capillaries and venules.
Treatment	**Nasal packing, cautery**, and **estrogens** may be tried to control recurrent epistaxis; significant visceral AV malformations may require embolization.
Discussion	Hereditary hemorrhagic telangiectasia, or Osler-Weber-Rendu syndrome, is inherited as an **autosomal-dominant trait**. Telangiectasias may first be seen during adolescence and then increase in incidence with age, peaking between the ages of 45 and 60 years. AV fistulas may present with hemoptysis, indicating high morbidity.
Atlas Link	UCV2 MC-145

OSLER–WEBER–RENDU SYNDROME

ID/CC	A **45-year-old woman** visits her dermatologist complaining of **painful, blistering skin lesions over her back, chest, and arms that break down and leave denuded skin areas**.
HPI	Over the past few years she has had **large recurrent aphthous ulcers in the mouth**. She was not taking any drugs before her symptoms developed.
PE	**Large aphthous ulcers** seen over oral and vaginal mucosa; **vesiculobullous skin lesions** seen in **various stages**; vertical pressure over bullae leads to **lateral extension** ("BULLA SPREAD SIGN"); skin over bullae **peels like that of a "hot tomato"** (NIKOLSKY'S SIGN).
Labs	Indirect immunofluorescence test to detect antibodies in serum shows presence of IgG antibodies.
Gross Pathology	Fresh vesicle is selected for biopsy.
Micro Pathology	Lesions show **loss of cohesion of epidermal cells** (ACANTHOLYSIS) that produces clefts directly above basal cell layer; Tzanck smear of material from floor of a bulla reveals acantholytic cells that are round with large hyperchromatic nuclei and homogeneous cytoplasm; **direct immunofluorescence** reveals **characteristic IgG intercellular staining** and **deposits**.
Treatment	Steroids are mainstay of therapy; cytotoxic drugs (cyclophosphamide).
Discussion	Pemphigus vulgaris, an intraepidermal blistering disease of the skin and mucous membranes, usually appears in individuals in the third to fifth decade of life. The blisters result from loss of adhesion between epidermal cells caused by the production of autoantibodies that are directed against keratinocyte cell surface proteins; loss of cell-cell contact between desmosomes (which are sites of attachment for epidermal cells) has been demonstrated by electron microscopy. Untreated pemphigus vulgaris is often fatal.
Atlas Links	UCV1 PM-P1-043 　　 UCV2 MC-019

ID/CC	A 17-year-old girl presents with a **scaly rash** on her **trunk**.
HPI	Three weeks ago, she noticed a small scaly rash on her neck that progressed in about a week to involve the trunk and upper extremities. Aside from the rash, she is asymptomatic. She is sexually active.
PE	VS: normal. PE: crop of **oval, erythematous, scaly maculopapular lesions** on trunk, neck, and proximal extremities in a **"Christmas tree" distribution**.
Labs	RPR/VDRL non-reactive; ELISA for HIV negative.
Gross Pathology	Biopsy specimen shows **superficial perivascular dermatitis**.
Treatment	Treat with **moisturizers** and **antipruritic lotions; topical steroids** or **oral antihistamines** rarely required; **ultraviolet B light** used to relieve pruritus in resistant cases; provide reassurance, since disease is **benign and self-limited**, and **recurrence** is **uncommon**.
Discussion	**Pityriasis rosea** is a common skin rash with the highest incidence in young adults and teenagers. The disease is twice as common in women as in men. In most cases, the initial lesion is a 1- to 10-cm, oval maculopapular lesion, called a **"herald patch,"** that is commonly found on the trunk or neck. Pityriasis rosea is a clinical diagnosis; it is important to differentiate the disease from **secondary syphilis, tinea versicolor, psoriasis**, and **drug reactions**.

ID/CC	A 40-year-old male comes to a dermatology outpatient clinic with an extensive, mildly pruritic, and chronic skin rash.
HPI	**It improves during the summer and markedly worsens in cold weather.** The patient was previously diagnosed by an orthopedic surgeon with **distal interphalangeal joint arthropathy**.
PE	Multiple **salmon-colored plaques** with **overlying silvery scales** seen over back and extensor aspects of upper and lower limbs; on removing scale, **underlying pinpoint bleeding capillaries** seen (AUSPITZ SIGN); lesions seen along scratch marks (KOEBNER PHENOMENA); **pitting of nails** with occasional onycholysis seen.
Imaging	XR, hands: asymmetric degenerative changes involving the distal interphalangeal joints, with **"pencil-in-cup"** deformity.
Micro Pathology	Skin biopsy reveals markedly thickened stratum corneum with layered zones of parakeratosis (retention of nuclei); markedly hyperplastic epidermis with elongation of rete projections; collections of PMNs within the stratum corneum (MUNRO'S MICROABSCESSES); **marked degree of epidermal hyperplasia with little inflammatory infiltrate** (characteristic microscopic finding).
Treatment	Exposure to sunlight. The following have been used either alone or in combination: occlusive dressings, tar ointment, dithranol, PUVA, topical steroids, and cytotoxic drugs such as methotrexate.
Discussion	Psoriasis is a hereditary condition that is characterized by well-defined plaques covered by silvery scales. Lesions are most commonly seen in an extensor distribution, but the nails, scalp, palms, and soles may also be involved; arthritis of the distal interphalangeal joint may be seen in 20% of cases. Parenteral corticosteroids are contraindicated owing to the possibility of inducing pustular lesions.
Atlas Links	UCV2 IM2-008A, IM2-008B, IM2-008C

DERMATOLOGY

ID/CC	A **40-year-old female presents** with an extremely painful **ulcer** on her left **calf**.
HPI	The lesion appeared a month ago as a **small boil** after the patient hurt herself. It then became progressively larger until it cracked open 2 days ago. The patient reports a history of **ulcerative colitis**, which was diagnosed several years ago and managed effectively with steroid enemas and oral sulfasalazine.
PE	VS: normal. PE: 10- by 10-cm deep **ulcer with violaceous border** overhanging ulcer bed; no lymphadenopathy; good distal pulses palpable (vs. arterial insufficiency ulcer); neurological exam normal.
Labs	No growth demonstrated on Gram stain and culture of wound swab; **skin biopsy diagnostic**.
Micro Pathology	Skin biopsy reveals hyperkeratosis; dermal perivascular round cell infiltration, and mixed infiltrate (neutrophils, lymphocytes, macrophages) extending to the subcutaneous plane.
Treatment	Systemic **steroids** (oral prednisone or IV pulse methylpred-nisone) and **immunosuppressive** therapy (cyclosporine or tacrolimus); antibiotics for secondary infection and narcotic analgesics for pain.
Discussion	Commonly associated conditions include **inflammatory bowel disease** and **leukemia** or **preleukemic states** (usually myelocytic leukemia or monoclonal gammopathies). Most cases occur in the fourth or fifth decades of life, with females affected slightly more often than males.

PYODERMA GANGRENOSUM

ID/CC	A 40-year-old white male presents with a **scaly, mildly pruritic rash over the face and scalp**.
HPI	He reports that the rash is **aggravated by humidity, scratching, emotional stress, and seasonal changes**. He tested **HIV positive** last year and has since maintained a good CD4+ count without any antiretroviral therapy.
PE	VS: normal. PE: interspersed thick **adherent crusts and scales** overlying areas of **greasy, yellow-red inflamed skin** involving the **scalp, forehead, nasolabial folds**, and **chest**.
Treatment	Maintain **good hygiene; medicated shampoo; topical hydrocortisone lotion** or ketoconazole cream.
Discussion	A papulosquamous skin rash involving areas rich in sebaceous glands; seborrheic dermatitis is thought to result from an abnormal host immune response toward a common skin commensal, *Pityrosporum ovale*. Various drugs (haloperidol, lithium, methyldopa, cimetidine) may worsen the condition. It is also commonly found in patients suffering from parkinsonism and in those recovering from an acute MI.

SEBORRHEIC DERMATITIS

ID/CC	A 19-year-old **black male** complains of **unsightly white** (depigmented) **patches** on his knees and elbows (bony prominences).
HPI	He has no history of associated **pruritus** or **discomfort**. The first patch appeared over the left elbow a few months ago, and the process has been **progressive** since then.
PE	PE: flat, well-demarcated areas of **depigmentation** on face (perioral or periocular), elbows, knees, and neck and in skin folds; sites of recent skin trauma are also seen to have **undergone depigmentation** (KOEBNER'S PHENOMENON); **most hairs within vitiliginous patch are white**.
Micro Pathology	**Absent melanin pigment** on skin biopsy stain with ferric ferricyanide; **absence of melanocytes** on electron microscopy.
Treatment	No established satisfactory treatment exists, although sunscreens protect and limit the tanning of normally pigmented skin. A promising approach is oral psoralen (a photosensitizing drug) followed by exposure to artificial long-wave ultraviolet light (UVA); potent fluorinated topical steroids may also be helpful. Generalized vitiligo may be treated by depigmentation of normal skin.
Discussion	Vitiligo usually appears in otherwise-healthy persons, but several systemic disorders occur more often in patients with vitiligo, including thyroid disease (e.g., hyperthyroidism, Graves' disease, and thyroiditis), Addison's disease, pernicious anemia, alopecia areata, uveitis, and diabetes mellitus. Precipitating factors such as illness, emotional stress, or physical trauma are often associated with its onset. The disease may be inherited as an **autosomal-dominant trait** with incomplete penetrance and variable expression. Most studies, however, point to an **autoimmune** basis (circulating complement-binding anti-melanocyte antibodies have been detected).
Atlas Link	UCV2 MC-153

ID/CC	An obese **44-year-old female** complains of **irritability** and excessive weight gain (40 kg) over the past 3 years and requests medical weight-loss therapy.
HPI	On careful questioning, she also reports **easy bruising, oligomenorrhea, weakness, and increased hair growth** in various areas of her body.
PE	VS: hypertension (BP 180/110). PE: facial acne; **truncal obesity** with thin extremities; **buffalo hump** and plethoric **moon facies; hirsutism**; wide, purple abdominal and lower leg **striae**.
Labs	UA: 3+ **glycosuria. Elevated fasting blood sugar; elevated plasma cortisol**; high ACTH. Lytes: **hypokalemia**. CBC: leukopenia. **Dexamethasone suppression test** fails to suppress hypercortisolism.
Imaging	XR, plain: **generalized osteoporosis**.
Gross Pathology	Pituitary adenoma; bilateral **adrenocortical hyperplasia**.
Micro Pathology	Pituitary: benign basophilic adenoma with Crook's hyalinization.
Treatment	Surgical removal of pituitary adenoma (transsphenoidal adenectomy) or pituitary irradiation along with adjunct medical therapy.
Discussion	Cushing's syndrome comprises the manifestations of hypercortisolism regardless of its cause; causes include excess glucocorticoid administration, paraneoplastic processes (ECTOPIC), ACTH production, adrenal lesions that produce excess cortisol, and pituitary lesions that produce excess ACTH (CUSHING'S DISEASE).
Atlas Links	UCV2 IM1-019A, IM1-019B, IM1-019C, IM1-019D

ENDOCRINOLOGY

ID/CC	A 40-year-old **woman** is seen in the outpatient clinic with complaints of sudden-onset **painful neck swelling**.
HPI	Prior to this she had a **sore throat, malaise, and fever**. Pain over the thyroid area radiates to the ears and is worse on swallowing.
PE	VS: fever; tachycardia. PE: fine **tremors** of tongue and fingers of outstretched hands; firm, exquisitely **tender, diffuse, mildly enlarged goiter** palpable; nonfirm nodularity felt; no cervical lymphadenopathy; no ophthalmopathy (distinguishes from Graves').
Labs	**CBC: elevated leukocytes. Elevated ESR** (characteristic); elevated free T_3 and T_4 levels and resin uptake (seen only during early stages due to follicular disruption and hormone release; later transient hypothyroidism may ensue; rarely, permanent hypothyroidism results); depressed TSH; markedly **reduced radioactive iodine uptake** (key diagnostic feature and used for differentiating it from Graves' disease).
Imaging	Nuc: poorly visualized thyroid gland.
Gross Pathology	Diffusely enlarged thyroid gland; involved areas are firm and yellow against the normal uninvolved brown thyroid substance.
Micro Pathology	Early lesions include **disruption of thyroid follicles with a neutrophilic infiltrate and formation of microabscesses**; subsequently, **multinucleated giant cells** may be seen surrounding colloid fragments, resembling granulomas.
Treatment	**Propranolol and analgesics** for symptomatic relief are generally adequate. The condition is **self-limiting**, lasting 6 to 8 weeks. Severe cases may require **prednisone** therapy; permanent hypothyroidism may result on rare occasions, in which case hormone replacement is required. **Antithyroid drugs are not indicated**.
Discussion	De Quervain's thyroiditis, or subacute **painful** thyroiditis, is the most common cause of severe thyroid pain and tenderness; it is most common in **women 20 to 50 years** of age and shows an association with **HLA-B35**. Its exact etiology is unknown, but viral causes have been implicated.

ID/CC	An **8-year-old** black male is brought to his pediatrician because of a 4-kg **weight loss** over a period of 3 months.
HPI	His mother says that he has also been complaining of **excessive thirst, hunger, and urination** (POLYDIPSIA, POLYPHAGIA, POLYURIA). The patient also reports **waking up several times during the night to urinate** (NOCTURIA).
PE	**Thinly built** male child with an otherwise-normal physical exam.
Labs	**Elevated fasting blood sugar** (180 mg/dL); elevated postprandial blood sugar (270 mg/dL). UA: **glycosuria. Islet cell antibodies** and **anti-insulin antibodies in serum**; elevated glycosylated hemoglobin (**hemoglobin A$_{1C}$**).
Micro Pathology	Decreased number of pancreatic β islets with hyalinization, fibrosis, and lymphocytic infiltration.
Treatment	**Insulin** (type I diabetics do not have circulating insulin and require exogenous insulin to **prevent diabetic ketoacidosis**), sugar-restricted diet.
Discussion	Previously known as **insulin-dependent diabetes mellitus (IDDM)**, diabetes mellitus type I typically arises before age 20 and is caused by **autoimmune** (T-cell) destruction of β cells. It may be triggered by coxsackievirus B4, mumps, or other viruses in individuals with a genetic predisposition, and it is linked to **chromosome 6-HLA-DR3 or -DR4**. Close-to-normal values of **glycosylated hemoglobin** reflect good long-term control of blood sugar levels. The main causes of death (in descending order) are myocardial infarction, renal failure, cerebrovascular disease, and infection. Other manifestations include **blindness, retinopathy, peripheral neuropathy**, and **gangrene** of extremities.

DIABETES MELLITUS TYPE I (JUVENILE ONSET)

ID/CC	An **obese 55-year-old** white male complains of increasing **thirst** and **excessive appetite**.
HPI	He also complains of **increased urinary volume**, weight loss, and weakness over the past several months together with burning and **tingling sensations** in a **stocking-glove distribution** (suggesting peripheral neuropathy). His father was diabetic with a history of leg amputation and kidney failure.
PE	VS: hypertension (BP 150/95). PE: **"dot-blot" hemorrhages, exudates, and microaneurysms** on funduscopic exam; muscle atrophy in hips and thighs; diminished dorsalis pedis and tibialis pulses bilaterally.
Labs	**Elevated glycosylated hemoglobin** (HEMOGLOBIN A_{1c}). UA: **glycosuria**. Elevated fasting serum glucose (HYPERGLYCEMIA).
Micro Pathology	Amyloidosis; hyaline atherosclerosis; nodular hyaline masses (KIMMELSTIEL–WILSON NODULES) in glomerulus.
Treatment	Diet and exercise; oral hypoglycemic agents; insulin as needed.
Discussion	Previously known as **non-insulin-dependent diabetes mellitus**, diabetes mellitus type II is a metabolic disease involving carbohydrates and lipids caused by peripheral **resistance to insulin**. Although patients with type II diabetes mellitus are not prone to developing diabetic ketoacidosis, they can develop **nonketotic hyperosmolar coma** if their blood glucose is drastically elevated. Sequelae of type I and type II diabetes mellitus include peripheral vascular disease, coronary artery disease, stroke, diabetic nephropathy, diabetic neuropathy, nonhealing skin ulcers, and delayed wound healing with increased risk of infection.

ID/CC	A **45-year-old woman** presents with a **swelling in the anterior portion of her neck**.
HPI	She also complains of **slowed speech, easy fatigability,** and **cold intolerance.** She is known to have **rheumatoid arthritis**, for which she is taking NSAIDs.
PE	**Puffy face; dry skin; coarse hair; swelling of thyroid gland** in anterior portion of neck; swelling is mobile with deglutition but not with protrusion of tongue; thyroid has rubbery consistency; right lobe more enlarged than left; swan neck deformity of left ring finger; ulnar deviation of fingers of both hands.
Labs	T_3, T_4 low; TSH high; **antithyroglobulin antibodies** and **antimicrosomal antibodies** (ANTITHYROID PEROXIDASE ANTIBODIES) detected by ELISA.
Imaging	Nuc: decreased radioactive iodine uptake (RAIU).
Gross Pathology	Diffuse, moderate enlargement of thyroid gland; cut surface is light gray and appears similar to a lymph node.
Micro Pathology	Biopsy shows massive infiltration by lymphocytes and plasma cells; normal follicles not present; scant colloid; eosinophilic **Hürthle cell** degeneration seen.
Treatment	Replacement therapy with **levothyroxine (T_4).**
Discussion	Hashimoto's thyroiditis is often associated with other autoimmune diseases, including systemic lupus erythematosus, pernicious anemia, Sjögren's syndrome, and chronic hepatitis; it has a genetic association with HLA-DR5 (goitrous form) and HLA-DR3 (atrophic form). Thyrotoxicosis may be seen early in the course of this **autoimmune disease** owing to inflammatory disruption of thyroid follicles (HASHITOXICOSIS).

HASHIMOTO'S THYROIDITIS

ID/CC	A 24-year-old white female comes to her family doctor because of **weight loss** despite having a **good appetite**; she also complains of increasing **anxiety**.
HPI	She admits to having frequent bouts of **diarrhea**, reduced sleep capacity, **heat intolerance**, sweaty palms, **palpitations, tremors**, and **menstrual irregularity**.
PE	VS: **tachycardia**. PE: tremors of outstretched hand; **warm, moist skin; right lobe of thyroid palpably enlarged; left lobe not palpable**; no evidence of retrosternal goiter; no cervical lymphadenopathy.
Labs	**Increased T$_4$** (TOTAL PLASMA THYROXINE); increased resin triiodothyronine uptake (RT$_3$U); **decreased plasma TSH**.
Imaging	XR, soft tissue: no calcification in area of thyroid. CXR: no mediastinal mass. Nuc: **hyperfunctioning hot** (increased uptake) thyroid **nodule** with **decreased uptake in surrounding tissue and right other lobe** (due to atrophy of remainder of gland secondary to feedback inhibition of TSH).
Gross Pathology	Smooth, rounded, well-circumscribed single mass in right lobe of thyroid gland; no areas of hemorrhage or necrosis; remainder of gland atrophic.
Micro Pathology	No signs of atypia; follicular stroma with abundant, normal-appearing colloid.
Treatment	Treat thyrotoxicosis with **propranolol** and antithyroid medications (e.g., propylthiouracil and methimazole); ablation of adenoma by either radioactive iodine or surgery.
Discussion	Plummer's nodule is a variant of toxic nodular goiter in which hyperthyroidism is caused by overproduction of thyroid hormone by a single thyroid adenoma known as **toxic adenoma**.
Atlas Link	UCV1 PG-P1-054

ID/CC	A 46-year-old white male visits his family doctor complaining of **impotence** and **fatigue** over the past year along with **decreased peripheral vision**.
HPI	He also complains of **decreased appetite** and **cold intolerance**. Last week, he scratched both sides of his car while driving through an alley.
PE	VS: **hypotension** (due to decreased ACTH). PE: pallor; **bitemporal hemianopsia** on visual field testing; optic atrophy; loss of axillary and pubic hair; increasingly sparse beard; smooth, dry skin; **testicular atrophy**.
Labs	Lytes: hyponatremia. **Low FSH, LH, TSH, and ACTH**; correspondingly low T_3, T_4, cortisol, estrogen, and testosterone; hypoglycemia.
Imaging	CT/MR: **pituitary mass** compressing optic chiasm. XR, skull: widening of sella turcica.
Gross Pathology	Compression of optic chiasm and hypothalamus by pituitary adenoma; may undergo infarction; atrophy of thyroid, testes, and adrenals.
Micro Pathology	Adenoma of chromophobe cells with abundant cytoplasm lacking granules.
Treatment	Surgical resection (transsphenoidal adenectomy) and hormone replacement (glucocorticoids, levothyroxine [T_4], testosterone).
Discussion	The most common cause of hypopituitarism is **adenoma** compressing the anterior pituitary. Other common causes are **ischemic necrosis** of the anterior pituitary in postpartum females (SHEEHAN'S SYNDROME), pituitary surgery/radiation, and, in children, **craniopharyngiomas**.

ENDOCRINOLOGY

HYPOPITUITARISM

ID/CC A 6-year-old boy is brought in for a pediatric consultation due to a hoarse voice, **growth retardation**, and developmental delay.

HPI The boy's mother describes a **prolonged gestation** and a birth weight of 4.5 kg. The boy has had problems at school owing to a short attention span, sleeping in class, and **mental sluggishness**.

PE Dry, **yellowish skin**; wide-based ataxic gait; **large tongue** (MACROGLOSSIA); muscular atrophy; **short stature** for age; broad nose; **umbilical hernia**; puffy eyes (due to myxedema) and wide epicanthal distance; slow relaxation of tendon reflexes; thin, brittle hair; **protuberant abdomen**; weak, hoarse voice.

Labs Elevated TSH; low T_3 and T_4.

Imaging XR, plain: absence of some ossification centers; coxa vara (DECREASED FEMORAL ANGLE); delayed epiphyseal development.

Gross Pathology Enlarged thyroid gland; **myxedema**; failure of sexual organs to develop properly.

Treatment **Levothyroxine replacement.**

Discussion **Congenital hypothyroidism** in an infant or child leads to **irreversible mental retardation**; it is caused by lack of iodine, thyroid developmental defects, radioactive iodine exposure during pregnancy, autoimmune disorders, and drugs. Protean manifestations include neuromuscular impairment, short stature (dwarfism), cardiovascular symptoms, and **sexual retardation**; it can be **mistaken for Down's syndrome** with grave consequences. All states in the United States currently require neonatal screening for hypothyroidism, galactosemia, and phenylketonuria.

HYPOTHYROIDISM—CONGENITAL

ID/CC	A 48-year-old white female complains of progressive **weakness, lethargy**, and **cold intolerance**.
HPI	She also complains of **weight gain, constipation, coarsening of her facial features**, hair loss, and increasing **hoarseness** in her voice. She adds that her periods have become irregular and heavy. Her husband notes that she has become increasingly forgetful and **depressed**.
PE	VS: bradycardia. PE: coarse facial features; periorbital edema; yellowish skin that is rough, cold, and dry; **brittle, thinning hair; loss of hair of outer third of eyebrows**; cardiomegaly; enlarged tongue; **delayed recovery phase** of Achilles tendon reflex.
Labs	Low T_3 and T_4; elevated TSH; elevated serum cholesterol.
Imaging	Nuc: low radioactive iodine uptake (RAIU) by the thyroid.
Micro Pathology	Myxoid degeneration of connective tissue, harboring isolated areas of atrophic follicle; lymphocytic infiltrate seen if Hashimoto's thyroiditis is the etiology.
Treatment	**Levothyroxine (T_4)** replacement.
Discussion	The most common causes of hypothyroidism are **Hashimoto's thyroiditis** and hyperthyroidism that has been treated with **surgery** or **radioactive iodine**; it may be **primary** (TSH is high) or **secondary** (low production of TSH by pituitary).

HYPOTHYROIDISM—PRIMARY

ID/CC	A **7-year-old male** is brought to a physician for an evaluation of **precocious puberty**.
HPI	He has a history of **severe headaches and visual blurring**.
PE	**Fully developed secondary sexual characteristics** (Tanner stage IV); **paralysis of upward gaze** (PARINAUD SYNDROME); convergence retraction nystagmus; funduscopy reveals **bilateral papilledema**; wide-based gait.
Labs	Normal lab parameters.
Imaging	MR, head: **obstructive hydrocephalus and brightly enhancing mass in region of pineal gland**.
Micro Pathology	Microscopic pathology reveals tumor to be of **germ cell origin** (GERMINOMA).
Treatment	Neurosurgery, removal of the tumor or shunt placement, and radiation therapy are the mainstays of treatment.
Discussion	Pineal region tumors include **pineocytomas and pineoblastomas** derived from the pineal parenchymal cells as well as **teratomas and germinomas**; precocious puberty occurs in young males, primarily as a result of **destruction of the pineal gland by a germinoma**. Pinealomas may produce hypothalamic hormone deficiency, leading to hypopituitarism or diabetes insipidus.

ID/CC	A 33-year-old white female presents with **menstrual cycle irregularity** with long periods of **amenorrhea** and **milky nipple discharge** (GALACTORRHEA).
HPI	Further questioning discloses that she has also **been unable to conceive**.
PE	VS: BP normal. PE: no gynecological masses palpable; pelvic exam normal.
Labs	Hyperprolactinemia; reduced LH and estradiol.
Imaging	MR: enhancing pituitary microadenoma (< 10 mm); deviation of pituitary stalk.
Treatment	**Bromocriptine** (dopamine analog) to inhibit prolactin synthesis and release (and to reduce size of large tumors); consider transsphenoidal surgery in patients whose tumors remain large despite bromocriptine therapy, in those who cannot tolerate dopamine agonists, and in psychiatric patients who require dopamine antagonists.
Discussion	Prolactinoma is the most common type of pituitary adenoma. Hypothalamic GnRH is suppressed by excessive prolactin secretion by the tumor, and thus LH and estradiol are reduced. In **males**, it presents with **headache, impotence**, and **visual disturbance**. Pathologic hyperprolactinemia can also be caused by the interruption of hypothalamic dopaminergic suppression of pituitary prolactin release (e.g., suprasellar masses, pituitary stalk section, and drugs such as haloperidol, phenothiazines, and reserpine). Thus, mild hyperprolactinemia does not always signify the presence of a neoplasm. Elevated estrogen (stimulates lactotrophs) and renal insufficiency are additional causes of hyperprolactinemia.

ENDOCRINOLOGY

ID/CC A 40-year-old woman complains of an unsightly, **progressively increasing neck swelling** and intermittent shortness of breath.

HPI She has noticed unusually **engorged neck veins** and has recently developed **difficulty swallowing solids** (DYSPHAGIA) and **loud snoring** (STRIDOR) while sleeping. There are **no symptoms of hypothyroidism or hyperthyroidism**. She uses iodized salt (iodine deficiency produces endemic goiter).

PE PE: anterior, **irregularly surfaced swelling that moves with deglutition** (MULTINODULAR GOITER); percussion over sternum is dull (due to retrosternal extension of goiter); **suffusion of face with marked dyspnea when patient raises both arms** overhead for a few seconds (due to tracheal compression); **no tremors or eye signs**; no cervical adenopathy.

Labs T_3, T_4 normal; **TSH elevated**; thyroid autoantibodies absent.

Imaging CXR: **retrosternal extension** of the goiter, producing tracheal compression and deviation. US/CT: **diffuse multinodularity**.

Gross Pathology Resected **thyroid grossly enlarged**; surface **covered by nodules of varying sizes**.

Micro Pathology Follicles **distended with colloid**; follicle lining cells flattened; degenerative changes present in between nodules.

Treatment **Subtotal thyroidectomy**; **thyroxine** subsequently administered to **suppress** TSH levels and prevent recurrence.

Discussion The cause of enlargement of the thyroid is most often unknown; known causes include **iodine deficiency** (in endemic areas), **ingestion of goitrogens** (e.g., cabbage, cassava), water pollutants, or **defects** in the synthesis or transport of hormone. In addition to tracheal compression and dysphagia, substernal goiters can also cause phrenic or recurrent laryngeal nerve palsies, esophageal varices, and Horner's syndrome.

Atlas Links UCVI PG-P1-060, PM-P1-060

ID/CC	A 50-year-old **female** presents with a **nodule in the front of her neck** that she first noticed 1 month ago.
HPI	She notes that the nodule has grown, but she does not complain of any symptoms suggestive of a hyperthyroid or hypothyroid state. She consumes iodized salt. She works as an **x-ray technician** (radiation exposure).
PE	**Firm, nontender nodule** in anterior portion of neck, mobile with deglutition; anterior cervical lymphadenopathy; no tremors, sweating, pretibial/pedal myxedema, or exophthalmos.
Labs	**Normal thyroid function tests**; normal thyroid hormone levels.
Imaging	XR, neck: stippled calcification. Nuc: **cold nodule**. US: **solid nodule**.
Gross Pathology	Nodule can range in size from microscopic to several centimeters with invasive margins; may be sclerotic or partly cystic.
Micro Pathology	FNA: **psammoma bodies**; lymphocytes; large pink follicular cells with **empty-appearing nuclei** ("Orphan Annie" nuclei) and eosinophilic intranuclear inclusions.
Treatment	Ipsilateral lobectomy and exploration of regional lymph nodes; follow up levels of serum thyroglobulin; levothyroxine suppression.
Discussion	**Ionizing radiation** is a predisposing factor for the development of **papillary carcinoma** of the thyroid. Papillary carcinoma spreads via the lymphatics and may present with only cervical lymphadenopathy and an occult primary. In contrast, follicular and sporadic medullary carcinomas commonly metastasize via the bloodstream. Of all histologic variants of thyroid cancer **(papillary, follicular, anaplastic, medullary)**, papillary carcinoma carries the best prognosis and anaplastic carcinoma the worst. Medullary carcinoma of the thyroid is derived from **parafollicular cells** (C cells) and is most commonly sporadic, but it may also occur in familial forms with multiple endocrine neoplasia (MEN) types IIA and IIB.
Atlas Link	UCV1 PM-P1-061

ENDOCRINOLOGY

ID/CC A 5-year-old **Asian** female develops **sudden**, acute **pain** and **loss of vision** in the right eye after watching a series of family slides in a **dark room**.

HPI She had been complaining of seeing **"halos" around lights** at night.

PE Injection (due to vasodilation) of ciliary and conjunctival blood vessels; **hazy cornea**; loss of peripheral vision; **markedly elevated intraocular pressure**; shallow anterior chamber with peripheral iridocorneal contact by slit-lamp exam; pupils mid-dilated and unresponsive to light and accommodation; hyperemic and edematous optic nerve bed on funduscopic exam.

Gross Pathology Pathologically narrow anterior chamber; eye hyperopic and **rock-hard** in consistency; synechia formation; Schlemm's canal may be blocked.

Micro Pathology Degeneration and fibrosis of trabeculae.

Treatment Analgesics, IV acetazolamide; topical beta-blockers; steroids; pilocarpine; **laser iridotomy**.

Discussion Acute angle-closure glaucoma is characterized by a sudden increase in intraocular pressure that may be **precipitated by mydriatics** and upon leaving **dark environments** for well-lit areas.

ID/CC   A 28-year-old **woman** presents with a sudden, severe attack of
         vertigo associated with nausea and vomiting.

HPI   Her symptoms begin and are aggravated when she looks toward
         the right. The attacks last less than 30 seconds. She has no
         history of hearing loss, ear discharge, tinnitus, trauma, pain, or
         restricted neck movement.

PE   Symptoms recur when her head is turned toward right; rotatory
         fatigable nystagmus with a linear component; no hearing loss or
         any other neurologic deficit.

Treatment Reassurance and positioning maneuvers designed to clear debris
           from the posterior canal.

Discussion Benign positional vertigo is sometimes seen after head injuries,
            ear operations, or infections of the middle ear; it is thought to
            be due to free-floating otoconial debris in the posterior semicir-
            cular canal. It typically abates spontaneously after a few weeks or
            months.

ID/CC A 35-year-old male seen after a roadside accident presents with a **persistent bloody but thin nasal discharge**.

HPI Directed questioning reveals that he has also **lost his sense of smell** since the accident.

PE Watery nasal discharge noted; **bilateral periorbital hematomas** ("black eye") seen; **anosmia** found on neurologic exam; remainder of physical exam normal; on placing a drop of nasal discharge on clean white gauze, **spreading yellow halo noted in addition to central blood stain** ("HALO SIGN"; due to presence of CSF).

Imaging CT, head: **fracture of cribriform plate**.

Treatment Antibiotics; head end elevated by 30 degrees; patient **advised not to blow his nose**; neurosurgical consult for possible repair of meninges.

Discussion Fractures of the base of the skull involve the anterior or middle cranial fossa. Those affecting the anterior fossa, as in this case, may cause nasal bleeding, periorbital hematomas, subconjunctival hemorrhages, CSF rhinorrhea, and cranial nerve injuries (CN I–CN V); **middle cranial fossa structures involving the petrous temporal bone may cause bleeding from the ear, CSF otorrhea, bruising of the ear over the mastoid** ("BATTLE SIGN"), **and cranial nerve injuries** (CN VII–CN VIII).

ID/CC A **50-year-old male** complains of **hearing loss and a whistling sound in his left ear** (TINNITUS).

HPI He claims to have pronounced **difficulty understanding speech** (out of proportion to hearing loss). He has also experienced occasional **vertigo**.

PE Left-sided **sensorineural deafness; Weber test lateralized toward right ear**; left-sided corneal reflex lost (CN V dysfunction).

Labs Pure-tone audiometry reveals sensorineural hearing loss; **discrimination of speech markedly reduced**; loudness recruitment absent; tone decay seen.

Imaging CT: left **cerebellopontine-angle tumor** suggestive of acoustic neuroma.

Gross Pathology **Encapsulated tumor** arising out of periphery of CN VIII (vestibular division) at cerebellopontine angle.

Micro Pathology **Spindle cells** with tightly interlaced pattern (ANTONI A) and **Verocay bodies**.

Treatment Surgical resection curative.

Discussion These benign tumors arise from the distal neurilemmal portion of the eighth nerve, usually from the vestibular division, and are correctly called schwannomas; they account for **80% of cerebellopontine tumors**. Acoustic neuromas can be successfully removed, but cranial nerve palsies such as CN VII nerve and deafness are common.

DEAFNESS—SENSORINEURAL

ID/CC A 30-year-old male complains of sudden-onset **dizziness, nausea, vomiting (nonprojectile), and loss of balance**.

HPI He also complains of headache and blurred vision (due to nystagmus). He has **chronic suppurative otitis media** (CSOM) of the right ear, for which he has taken treatment irregularly.

PE Patient lying on left ear and looking toward right ear; **conductive deafness**; Weber lateralized toward right ear) in right ear; horizontal spontaneous nystagmus toward left; purulent ear discharge from right ear; no neurologic deficits.

Imaging XR, mastoid area: **obliteration of mastoid air cells on right side**.

Treatment Surgical exploration of mastoid; antibiotics and vestibular suppressants.

Discussion Pyogenic inflammation of the labyrinth may result from acute otitis media, operations on the stapes, or preformed pathways such as fracture lines; in CSOM, cholesteatoma may cause erosion of the semicircular canals, exposing the labyrinth to infections. Meningitis is a serious complication of suppurative labyrinthitis.

ID/CC	A 45-year-old **obese** man presents with **excessive daytime sleepiness** that has progressively worsened over the past 3 years.
HPI	His wife complains that his **snoring** can be heard in the adjacent room and that he intermittently appears to stop breathing during the night. These **"no-breathing" episodes** last 30 to 90 seconds, and then, with a loud snort, he begins to breathe again. The patient also reports fatigue, forgetfulness, anxiety, **morning headaches**, and diminished sexual interest.
PE	VS: **mild hypertension** (140/90). PE: **short, thick neck; deviated nasal septum; pharyngeal crowding with enlarged, floppy uvula, high-arched palate and soft palate resting on base of tongue.**
Labs	Overnight pulse oximetry reveals **frequent episodes of arterial O_2 desaturation; polysomnography** (including EEG, ECG, eye movement, chin movement, air flow, chest and abdominal effort, SaO_2, snoring, and leg movement) **diagnostic.**
Treatment	**Weight loss**; avoidance of alcohol and sedatives; **nasal CPAP** or BiPAP; pharmacotherapy with protryptiline; **surgical interventions** include uvulopalatopharyngoplasty (UPPP).
Discussion	Pathophysiologically, nasopharyngeal crowding creates a critical subatmospheric pressure during inspiration that overcomes the ability of the airway dilator and abductor muscles to maintain airway patency. This causes apnea, leading to hypoxemia that eventually arouses the patient from sleep. In patients with obstructive sleep apnea, there is an **increased incidence** of **coronary events, CVAs,** and **right heart failure**.

OBSTRUCTIVE SLEEP APNEA

ID/CC	A **44-year-old black male** is referred to the ophthalmologist for evaluation of **progressive** and **painless diminution of vision**.
HPI	He has no known drug allergies and denies use of steroids.
PE	VS: normal. PE: ophthalmology exam reveals normal visual acuity with markedly **reduced peripheral field of vision**; **elevated intraocular pressure** on tonometry; **increased cup-to-disk ratio with optic atrophy** on ophthalmoscopy; wide open angle noted on gonioscopy.
Treatment	**Relief of intraocular hypertension** with topical beta-blockers (timolol), miotics (pilocarpine), or prostaglandin inhibitors with or without surgical procedures such as laser trabeculoplasty, trabeculotomy, goniotomy, and trabeculectomy.
Discussion	Open-angle glaucoma is the **most frequent cause of vision loss in the African-American population. Risk factors** include **diabetes, nearsightedness**, and **long-term steroid** use. People with **first-degree relatives** with glaucoma are at increased risk. Unfortunately, the disease is usually far advanced when symptoms are first noted. Prevention is through early detection with eye exams once every 2 years or more frequently for those at increased risk.

ID/CC   A **60-year-old male** complains of **progressively diminishing hearing acuity over the past few years**.

HPI   The patient's hearing loss is **bilateral** and is almost the **same for both ears**; he has no history of ear discharge, tinnitus, or trauma.

PE   Ability to distinguish between consonants markedly impaired; **air conduction exceeds bone conduction** (due to sensorineural hearing loss); audiometry reveals **bilateral hearing loss in higher-frequency range**.

Micro Pathology   Presbycusis is characterized by a loss of hair cells, atrophy of the spinal ganglion, altered endolymph production, and thickening of the basilar membrane with some neural degeneration.

Treatment   Counseling; some help could be obtained from a hearing aid.

Discussion   Presbycusis is a type of sensorineural hearing loss that results from the **aging process**; degenerative changes occur in the cells of the organ of Corti and nerve fibers. Deafness is bilateral and symmetrical, commonly **affecting the high tones**. Other types of presbycusis include strial, which starts in the fourth and sixth decades, is slowly progressive, and is characterized by good discrimination and by the presence of recruitment, a flat or descending audiogram, and patchy atrophy of the middle and apical turns of the stria. Cochlear deafness begins in middle age and is of the conductive variety, showing a downward slope on audiogram and absent pathologic findings. Both types of sensorineural loss can be avoided through use of protection in high-noise areas and monitoring of ototoxic drugs.

ID/CC	A 45-year-old male is seen with complaints of **blurring of vision while reading and performing similar tasks involving near vision**.
HPI	He complains that he has to hold the newspaper at an increasing distance in order to read it clearly. He has had no previous problems with his vision and has no history of diabetes or hypertension.
PE	**Amplitude of accommodation reduced**; convex lens reduced near-point distance, allowing patient to read comfortably and to engage in tasks requiring near vision.
Treatment	Convex lens glasses for work requiring near vision.
Discussion	Presbyopia is **natural loss of accommodation** due to **sclerosis of the lens substance**, which fails to adapt itself to a more spherical shape when the zonule is relaxed in the accommodation reflex. Presbyopia is seen in middle-aged patients (mean age 45 years).

ID/CC A 29-year-old woman visits a clinic with complaints of **visual blurring**.

HPI She also complains of **headaches** that are worse in the morning. She has been taking **oral contraceptives** for some time.

PE VS: BP normal. PE: patient is **obese**; funduscopy reveals presence of **papilledema**; no focal neurologic deficit noted; remainder of exam normal.

Labs LP: elevated opening pressure; CSF normal.

Imaging CT: ventricles normal, increased volume of subarachnoid spaces. Angio: rules out dural sinus thrombosis.

Treatment Stop oral contraceptives; advise diuretics and obesity-reducing measures. If medical treatment becomes inadequate, surgical options such as shunt placement are used.

Discussion Benign intracranial hypertension is primarily a disease of **obese females**; its etiology is unknown, although associations exist with the use of certain drugs (oral contraceptives, steroids, nalidixic acid, tetracycline) as well as with pregnancy, previous head injury, dural sinus thrombosis, and excessive vitamin A intake.

PSEUDOTUMOR CEREBRI

ID/CC	A **16-year-old male** is referred to an ophthalmologist for an evaluation of a **progressively constricting visual field**.
HPI	The boy complains that he sees as though he were looking **through a narrow tube**. Directed questioning reveals that he has a long-standing history of **night blindness** (due to loss of rods). His parents, although normal, had a **consanguineous marriage** and have a **family history of a visual disorder**.
PE	Funduscopy reveals **"bone spicule" pigmentation** in mid-periphery of fundus, waxy appearance of optic disk, and marked narrowing and attenuation of vessels; **field of vision shows concentric contraction** that is especially marked if illumination is reduced.
Labs	**Electroretinogram and electro-oculogram demonstrate reduced activity**.
Treatment	No satisfactory treatment; genetic counseling for prevention of the disease if the pattern of inheritance in a particular family can be traced.
Discussion	Retinitis pigmentosa is a **slow degenerative disease** of the retina that is always bilateral, begins in childhood, and results in blindness by middle or advanced age; the degeneration primarily affects the rods and the cones, particularly the rods, and commences in a zone near the equator, spreading both anteriorly and posteriorly. The condition may be associated with Laurence–Moon–Biedl syndrome (characterized by obesity, hypogenitalism, and mental subnormality), Refsum's disease (peripheral neuropathy, cerebellar ataxia, deafness, and ichthyosis due to a defect in phytanic acid metabolism), and abetalipoproteinemia. The condition is inherited as an autosomal-recessive trait in 40% of cases, as autosomal-dominant in 20%, and as X-linked in 5%.

ID/CC	An **18-month-old** boy presents with **diminished visual acuity** and a wandering right eye that his mother noticed while watching him play with his toys.
HPI	On directed history, the child admits to having **eye pain** at night.
PE	**White amaurotic "cat's eye" reflex** in right eye; deviation of right eye (STRABISMUS); **tenderness in eye** on gentle compression; **intraocular mass** on retinal examination.
Imaging	CT/MR, orbit: lobulated, hyperdense retrolental (behind lens) mass; no optic nerve compression.
Gross Pathology	Whitish mass behind lens.
Micro Pathology	Sheets of small, round blue cells with clusters of cuboidal or short columnar cells arranged around a central lumen (FLEXNER–WINTERSTEINER ROSETTES).
Treatment	Surgery.
Discussion	The **nonhereditary** variety of retinoblastoma appears as a single tumor; **hereditary** forms occur in early childhood and are often bilateral or multicentric. In hereditary cases, patients are at high risk for other cancers later in life (especially osteosarcoma). Cytogenetic studies reveal a **deletion on chromosome 13** (band 14 on long arm, Rb gene). Rb is a tumor suppressor gene; the loss of both allelic copies leads to malignancy (two-hit hypothesis).
Atlas Link	UCV1 PM-P1-073

ENT/OPHTHALMOLOGY

ID/CC	A 30-year-old male presents with sudden-onset **pain, redness, and tearing** in his left eye.
HPI	He also complains of **photophobia and blurred vision** in the left eye.
PE	VS: normal. PE: ophthalmologic exam reveals **conjunctival congestion, diminished visual acuity**, normal visual field, and pupillary miosis with normal reactivity; **aqueous flare with keratic precipitates** noted in anterior chamber on slit-lamp exam.
Labs	CBC: normal. ESR, ANA, RPR, VDRL, Lyme titer (to rule out systemic causes): normal.
Imaging	XR, chest and sacroiliac joints: normal.
Treatment	**Cycloplegics** (atropine) to relax pupillary sphincter and ciliary muscles; **topical corticosteroids**; occasionally immune suppression. Treat **underlying systemic illness**.
Discussion	Systemic disorders (sarcoidosis, SLE, ankylosing spondylitis, tuberculosis, syphilis) should be investigated as causes of uveitis.

ID/CC	A 33-year-old female complains of **increasing substernal pain and difficulty swallowing** liquids and solids (DYSPHAGIA) over the past several months.
HPI	She has lost 20 pounds in the past 3 months and has occasionally experienced acute substernal pain and **regurgitation of food into her mouth when lying down.**
PE	Unremarkable.
Labs	Esophageal manometry reveals aperistaltic esophagus; **increased lower esophageal sphincter pressure**; negative antinuclear antibodies (ANAs) (vs. scleroderma).
Imaging	UGI: **"rat-tailed" lower esophageal segment; dilatation;** uncoordinated peristalsis. EGD: gaping cavity filled with dirty fluid. CXR: air-fluid level in enlarged esophagus.
Gross Pathology	Massive dilatation of esophagus (due to defect in esophageal peristalsis and/or **impaired relaxation of lower esophageal sphincter** during swallowing).
Micro Pathology	Loss of number of ganglion cells in myenteric plexus (similar to Hirschsprung's disease of the colon).
Treatment	Heller's esophagocardiomyotomy; balloon dilatation; **botulinum toxin injection.**
Discussion	Primary **idiopathic** achalasia is a motility disorder of the esophagus due to **loss of ganglion cells in Auerbach's plexus.** Complications include esophageal **squamous cell carcinoma,** candidal esophagitis, diverticula, and/or aspiration pneumonia. Secondary achalasia may be caused by **Chagas' disease,** lymphoma, gastric carcinoma, or sarcoidosis.

ACHALASIA

ID/CC A **34-year-old woman** presents to the ER with complaints of **colicky abdominal pain, spiking fever, and vomiting**.

HPI She was diagnosed with **gallstones** on an abdominal ultrasound several weeks ago and is awaiting elective surgery.

PE VS: fever (39.4°C); tachycardia (HR 120); tachypnea (RR 24); mild hypotension (BP 94/60). PE: **toxic**-looking patient; **scleral icterus** noted; **marked RUQ tenderness** with mild hepatomegaly on abdominal exam.

Labs CBC: **leukocytosis. Markedly elevated direct bilirubin and alkaline phosphatase** with moderately elevated AST and ALT; normal albumin, PT, and PTT; **blood cultures** positive for *Escherichia coli*.

Imaging US, abdomen: **dilated common bile duct (CBD) with obstructing stone**. CT, abdomen: gallstones and stone in CBD with dilated intrahepatic bile ducts.

Treatment **NPO** with nasogastric suction; **IV antibiotics**; emergent endoscopic (interventional ERCP) or surgical **biliary tree decompression** followed by laparoscopic or open **cholecystectomy**.

Discussion Prolonged choledocholithiasis leads to suppurative cholangitis, which has a very high mortality rate.

ID/CC	A 50-year-old male presents with a long-standing history of **retrosternal burning, belching, and water brash**, especially after meals.
HPI	He is a **chronic smoker and alcoholic** and is under treatment for **gastroesophageal reflux dyspepsia**.
PE	Physical exam normal.
Labs	UGI endoscopy reveals linear streaks of red, velvety mucosa at gastroesophageal junction.
Imaging	Barium swallow: fine reticular pattern distal to an esophageal stricture; gastroesophageal reflux.
Gross Pathology	**Red, velvety mucosa in form of circumferential band and linear streaks around gastroesophageal junction**.
Micro Pathology	Mixture of **metaplastic gastric and intestinal-type columnar epithelial cells** (mucin-secreting and absorptive, respectively).
Treatment	Proton pump inhibitors, H_2 antagonists, and antacids; cessation of smoking and alcohol; careful endoscopic follow-up to detect esophageal cancer.
Discussion	Barrett's esophagus is marked by **metaplasia of the distal esophageal squamous epithelium to a columnar epithelium in response to prolonged injury**; long-standing esophageal reflux leads to inflammation and ulceration of squamous mucosa. Healing occurs through reepithelialization by pluripotent cells, which in the setting of low pH differentiates into the more resistant gastric (both cardiac and fundic) type or the specialized columnar (intestinal) type. Only the columnar type is of clinical importance. The most serious complication is the development of **adenocarcinoma**; hence, patients with Barrett's should undergo endoscopic surveillance every 2 to 3 years. Additional complications of Barrett's esophagus may include stricture formation and ulcerations.
Atlas Link	UCV1 PG-P1-077

GASTROENTEROLOGY

BARRETT'S ESOPHAGUS

ID/CC	A 40-year-old woman is seen with complaints of sudden-onset, progressively increasing **abdominal distention and pain** and **vomiting**.
HPI	The patient also complains of **visible abdominal and back veins** that appear while she is **standing** and **look like ropes**. In addition, she has observed **increasing swelling of her feet**. She has been taking **oral contraceptives** for a few years.
PE	Icterus; **pitting pedal edema**; markedly distended abdomen; dilated, tortuous veins over abdomen and back; **flow is from below upward** (due to hepatic vein and IVC obstruction); no jugular venous distention (therefore no right heart failure); **hepatojugular reflux absent**; fluid thrill but shifting dullness present (ascites); mildly tender **hepatomegaly and splenomegaly**.
Labs	CBC: leukocytosis. LFTs elevated; ascitic fluid **transudative**.
Imaging	US, abdomen: hepatosplenomegaly and ascites. US, Doppler: increased portal vein flow; **hepatic veins obstructed where they empty into the inferior vena cava**. IVC portovenography: confirms obstruction.
Gross Pathology	Thrombosis of hepatic vein where it drains into the inferior vena cava. Liver is swollen and reddish-purple and has a tense capsule.
Micro Pathology	Affected areas show severe centrilobular congestion and necrosis along with sinusoidal dilatation.
Treatment	Balloon angioplasty; thrombolytic therapy into hepatic veins; surgical removal or bypass of the obstruction; **cessation of oral contraceptives**; diuretics along with sodium and fluid restriction.
Discussion	Budd–Chiari syndrome occurs with conditions that predispose to thrombosis, e.g., polycythemia vera, pregnancy, postpartum states, use of oral contraceptives, paroxysmal nocturnal hemoglobinuria (PNH), and intra-abdominal cancers; membranous webs in the inferior vena cava may produce the obstruction. Untreated Budd–Chiari syndrome may progress to liver failure.

ID/CC	A 45-year-old male who has been diagnosed with **AIDS** presents with **pain on swallowing** (ODYNOPHAGIA) and mild **difficulty swallowing** (DYSPHAGIA).
HPI	These symptoms are markedly aggravated by the ingestion of acidic fluids.
PE	**Oral thrush**.
Labs	Culture of esophageal washings reveals *Candida albicans*.
Imaging	Esophagoscopy: small, raised **white or yellow plaques**.
Gross Pathology	Scattered yellowish-white plaques with occasional mucosal ulcers.
Micro Pathology	Cytologic examination of brushings reveals presence of yeast cells.
Treatment	Oral fluconazole.
Discussion	The current surge in candidal esophageal infections is due to AIDS and to post-organ-transplant immunosuppression therapy.
Atlas Links	UCV1 PG-P1-079, M-P1-079

CANDIDA ESOPHAGITIS

ID/CC	A 12-year-old white female, the daughter of **Norwegian** immigrants, complains of **diarrhea and flatulence**.
HPI	Her parents say she has suffered from weight loss despite the fact that she eats well. Her mother adds that her stool is **foul-smelling** and **greasy** (STEATORRHEA) with no blood or mucus.
PE	Pale and thin; xerosis (DRYNESS) and hyperkeratosis of skin (due to vitamin A malabsorption); vesicular rash on knees, elbows, and neck; **pruritus with erythematous base** (DERMATITIS HERPETIFORMIS); cheilosis (SCALING); ecchymoses (due to vitamin K malabsorption).
Labs	CBC: macrocytic, hypochromic anemia. Lytes: decreased potassium and calcium. **Elevated serum antigliadin** and **anti-endomysial antibodies**. Decreased serum cholesterol and albumin; prolonged PT; **abnormal d-xylose test**; positive Sudan stain for fecal fat.
Imaging	UGI/SBFT: loss of mucosal folds and **dilated jejunum**.
Micro Pathology	Hallmark **flattening and atrophy of mucosal villi** with basophilia and loss of nuclear polarity; lymphocytic and plasma cell infiltration of lamina propria.
Treatment	**Gluten-free diet**; glucocorticoids for refractory cases.
Discussion	Celiac disease is a disease of the small intestine that is due to **gluten** (gliadin) **hypersensitivity**. It is associated with HLA-DR3 and HLA-DQw2 and is characterized by varying degrees of **nutrient malabsorption**: iron, folate, fat-soluble vitamins (A, D, E, K). It is also known as **nontropical sprue, celiac sprue**, or gluten-sensitive enteropathy.
Atlas Links	UCVⅠ PM-P1-080A, PM-P1-080B

ID/CC	A **66-year-old Scandinavian** male comes to the doctor's office for an insurance physical complaining of increasing **fatigue, occasional indigestion, and diarrhea**.
HPI	He has been taking antacids for his dyspepsia.
PE	**Marked pallor; mild splenomegaly**.
Labs	CBC/PBS: **macrocytic anemia**, macro-ovalocytes, and hypersegmented neutrophils. Low vitamin B_{12} levels; elevated homocystine and methylmalonic acid; **Schilling test confirms vitamin B_{12} malabsorption** corrected with administration of intrinsic factor; **anti-parietal cell antibodies present; reduced gastric acid formation** (ACHLORHYDRIA); biopsy taken during endoscopy reveals **chronic atrophic gastritis** with no evidence of intestinal metaplasia. Endoscopy: thinning of mucosa and flattening of rugal fold seen more in fundus and body of stomach with **sparing of antrum**.
Gross Pathology	See labs.
Micro Pathology	Lymphocytes and plasma cell infiltrates in lamina propria; decreased number of glands.
Treatment	Parenteral administration of vitamin B_{12}; regular follow-up (chronic atrophic gastritis **predisposes to gastric carcinoma**).
Discussion	Pernicious anemia is characterized by chronic atrophic gastritis with achlorhydria and antibodies to parietal cells and intrinsic factor. The condition is more common among older patients (mean age of 60); these patients are predisposed to other autoimmune disorders, such as vitiligo, hypoparathyroidism, adrenal insufficiency, and thyroid disease.
Atlas Link	UCVI PM-P1-081

CHRONIC ATROPHIC GASTRITIS

ID/CC	A 45-year-old **alcoholic** male presents with **recurrent epigastric pain** that sometimes radiates to his back.
HPI	He also complains of **bulky, greasy, foul-smelling stool** (STEATORRHEA). He has **lost 10 pounds** over the past 3 months.
PE	**Epigastric pain** on deep palpation.
Labs	Quantitative estimation of fat in stool reveals **steatorrhea; elevated serum amylase and lipase levels**.
Imaging	XR, abdomen: **pancreatic calcification**. CT/US: **pancreatic atrophy and calcification**. ERCP: small stricture of pancreatic duct in head; distal pancreatic duct shows sacculation with intervening **short strictures** ("CHAIN OF LAKES").
Gross Pathology	**Scarred-down, fibrotic pancreas** with whitish areas of fatty necrosis and areas of **cystic cavitation**.
Micro Pathology	Pancreatic biopsy reveals presence of dilated ducts, fibrotic stroma, and atrophy of exocrine glands and islets (due to enzymatic fat necrosis).
Treatment	Pancreatic **enzyme replacement; low-fat diet**; surgery for relief of intractable pain.
Discussion	Chronic pancreatitis is a persistent inflammatory disease of the pancreas that is irreversible and causes pain and permanent impairment of endocrine and exocrine function. **Alcohol abuse is the most common cause in adults, cystic fibrosis in children.**
Atlas Links	UCV1 PG-P1-082, PM-P1-082

ID/CC	A 61-year-old white male in apparent good health has a routine annual physical exam that reveals a small rectal mass.
HPI	He has no major complaints except for intermittent, mild diarrhea.
PE	**Mobile, nonpainful rectal mass** on digital rectal exam with no evidence of bleeding; examination otherwise unremarkable.
Labs	CBC: **anemia** (Hb 9.2/Hct 26.9). **Hemoccult-positive stool.**
Imaging	Sigmoidoscopy/BE: multiple **pedunculated masses** in sigmoid and transverse colon.
Gross Pathology	Discrete mass lesions from colonic epithelium protruding into intestinal lumen; vast majority measure < 2 cm, although may reach up to 5 cm; may have stalk (PEDUNCULATED) or have a broad base (SESSILE); may be **tubular, villous,** or **tubulovillous.**
Micro Pathology	Frequent mitosis, cellular atypia, and loss of normal polarity in intestinal epithelium of glands.
Treatment	Colonoscopic biopsy and removal; repeat colonoscopy or barium enema for periodic surveillance.
Discussion	The **oncogene** associated with adenomatous polyposis coli is the **tumor suppressor gene** located on **chromosome 5.** The most common variety is adenomatous; the **risk of malignant transformation increases with size, villous** morphology, and the **familial** form of the disease (which has a 100% probability of becoming malignant).

GASTROENTEROLOGY

ID/CC	A 21-year-old female complains of **intermittent abdominal pain, mild, nonbloody diarrhea**, and anorexia of 2 years' duration.
HPI	She claims that during these episodes, she also has a fever; she adds that the pain is almost always confined to the **right lower abdomen** and is cramping in nature.
PE	Pallor; weight loss; **abdominal mass in right iliac fossa** (thickened bowel loop); **perianal fistulas**.
Labs	CBC: megaloblastic anemia; leukocytosis. **Guaiac positive**; stool exam reveals no parasites.
Imaging	BE: granulomatous colitis and **regional enteritis** involving multiple areas, most commonly ileum and ascending colon, with intervening segments of normal mucosa.
Gross Pathology	**Terminal ileum** (lesions most commonly seen in ileocecal area but can affect any part of the GI tract) shows lesions that have a **"cobblestone"** appearance; **discontinuous areas of inflammation, edema, and fibrosis** ("SKIP LESIONS"); toxic megacolon (thick intestinal wall, narrowed lumen).
Micro Pathology	**Chronic inflammatory involvement of submucosal layers of bowel wall** (TRANSMURAL INFLAMMATION), manifested mainly by lymphocytic infiltration with associated lymphoid hyperplasia and formation of noncaseating granulomas.
Treatment	**Antidiarrheal drugs and systemic glucocorticoids**; 5-aminosalicylic acid agents (e.g., sulfasalazine); azathioprine or mercaptopurine in patients with frequent exacerbations; **surgery** if patients develop severe malabsorption, symptomatic fistulas, or subacute intestinal obstruction.
Discussion	Complications of Crohn's disease include adhesions, ulcers, strictures, fissures, and fistulas. Extraintestinal manifestations may include arthritis, ankylosing spondylitis, sclerosing cholangitis, and uveitis. Crohn's disease patients also have a five- to six-fold increased risk of developing colon cancer; however, this risk is much lower than that associated with ulcerative colitis.

CROHN'S DISEASE

ID/CC	A 54-year-old white female complains of **colicky pain in the left lower abdomen** and **fever**.
HPI	She has had **frequent attacks of moderate pain** in the same area for several months and one episode of **bloody stools** without excessive mucus.
PE	VS: low-grade fever. PE: pallor; tenderness; rebound and guarding of left lower quadrant but normal stools; **sigmoid colon palpable, thickened, and tender**.
Labs	CBC: **normocytic, normochromic anemia; neutrophilic leukocytosis** with associated left shift (BANDEMIA). Stool culture reveals no pathogens.
Imaging	CT, abdomen: diverticular disease with **pericolonic inflammatory stranding**. BE (after acute phase): **"saw-toothed"** appearance.
Gross Pathology	Resected segment reveals external **outpouchings** up to 1 cm in diameter along colon between tenia coli **from lumen; small mucosal openings lead into pouches**.
Micro Pathology	A diverticulum sectioned along its axis shows **mucosa and submucosa herniating through a defect in the internal circular layer of muscularis**. Biopsy obtained during sigmoidoscopy reveals no malignancy.
Treatment	**High-fiber diet**; antibiotics for diverticulitis; surgical resection of severely involved segments.
Discussion	Diverticulitis is a condition of the colon in which the mucosa and submucosa herniate through the muscular layers of the colon to form outpouchings that may become obstructed with feces. The pathogenesis involves **increased intraluminal pressure** and **focal weakness** of the wall of the colon (near areas of nerve and vessel penetration alongside the taeniae coli). Outpouchings may become repeatedly inflamed, resulting in **abscess** formation, development of **fistulas** to adjoining organs, colonic obstruction, perforation, and sepsis. It is most commonly seen in the **sigmoid colon**.

DIVERTICULITIS

ID/CC	A **60-year-old** female presents with **lower abdominal discomfort**, **chronic constipation**, and **passage of bright red blood per rectum**.
HPI	She is a heavy smoker, and her diet contains a significant amount of greasy food and **little natural fiber**.
PE	VS: normal. PE: pallor; mild left lower abdominal tenderness with **palpable descending colon; guaiac-positive** stool on rectal exam.
Labs	CBC: normocytic, normochromic anemia. **Frank blood in stool; no leukocytes or epithelial cells** seen.
Imaging	Sigmoidoscopy: **multiple small outpouchings** in walls of **descending** and **sigmoid colon** without inflammation.
Gross Pathology	Multiple subcentimeter flasklike outpouchings alongside taeniae coli in walls of descending and sigmoid colon.
Micro Pathology	Thin-walled herniations of atrophic mucosa and compressed submucosa; hypertrophied circular layer of muscularis propria with prominent taeniae coli.
Treatment	**High dietary fiber**; supplement diet with soluble fiber and bulk-forming laxatives such as **psyllium**.
Discussion	Diverticuli are outpouchings in the colonic walls in which the arteries penetrate the muscularis layer to reach the mucosal wall, creating an inherently weak area. Most commonly found in the descending and sigmoid colon, diverticulosis is a disease of **Western industrialized society**, with a **low-fiber/high-fat diet** being a significant contributory factor. Complications include inflammation of the diverticuli (DIVERTICULITIS), significant lower GI bleeding, perforation, abscess formation, and colovesical fistula.
Atlas Links	⬛Ｕ Ｃ Ｖ Ｉ PG-P1-086, PM-P1-086

ID/CC	A 35-year-old female presents with **difficulty swallowing**.
HPI	She also complains of **retrosternal chest pain and heartburn**. She is not currently taking any medications, is a nonsmoker, and drinks alcohol only occasionally.
PE	VS: normal. PE: normal.
Labs	CBC: normal. ESR, ANA, RA factor: normal. ECG: normal.
Imaging	Esophagogram: irregular uncoordinated esophageal contractions (like a **giant corkscrew**). Esophageal manometry: lower part of esophagus demonstrates prolonged, **nonsequential, large-amplitude, repetitive contractions of simultaneous onset**.
Treatment	**Sublingual nitroglycerin** for acute attacks; anxiolytics and calcium channel blockers; H_2 blockers or proton pump inhibitors for associated GERD.
Discussion	Esophageal spasm is characterized by **uncoordinated esophageal muscle contractions** that do not propel food into the stomach. Esophageal spasm is seen in association with **advanced age, emotional stress**, collagen vascular disease, reflux esophagitis, esophageal obstruction, and irradiation esophagitis. Pain due to esophageal spasm **mimics angina**, which should be included in the differential diagnosis.

87 **ESOPHAGEAL SPASM**

ID/CC	A 47-year-old white **male** is brought by ambulance to the emergency room because of **massive, painless vomiting of bright red blood** (HEMATEMESIS) and shock.
HPI	He is a known homeless **alcoholic** who lives in the streets surrounding the hospital. His friend states that he has been drinking heavily for the past 2 months.
PE	VS: **tachycardia; hypotension**. PE: skin cold and clammy; **hard nodular hepatomegaly**; mild **splenomegaly**; spider nevi; caput medusae; clubbing; ascites, mild gynecomastia; bilaterally enlarged parotid glands.
Labs	CBC/PBS: normocytic, normochromic **anemia**. Low serum albumin; **elevated alkaline phosphatase; increased bilirubin, ALT, AST**.
Imaging	EGD: actively bleeding varices.
Gross Pathology	**Tortuous** and **dilated submucosal esophageal veins** secondary to shunting from **portal hypertension**; superficial ulceration, inflammation, and rupture.
Treatment	Restore blood volume, vasoconstrictors (e.g., vasopressin, somatostatin), balloon tamponade of varices followed by endoscopic sclerotherapy; splenorenal or other shunt if sclerotherapy fails.
Discussion	Esophageal varices are often silent until they rupture and are associated with a significant mortality rate. **Cirrhosis** is the most common cause, but other causes of portal hypertension may also be involved, including Budd–Chiari syndrome, tumor invasion of the portal vein, and metabolic diseases that alter liver sinusoids (e.g., amyloid).

ID/CC	A 35-year-old **obese** male **chronic smoker** presents with **heartburn**.
HPI	His heartburn **worsens** when bending and **lying down at night**, preventing him from sleeping; it is promptly **relieved with antacids**.
Labs	Continuous esophageal pH monitoring correlates symptoms with posture, meals, and reflux.
Imaging	UGI: small **hiatal hernia; spontaneous reflux** to mid-esophagus. EGD: erythema, friability, and erosions over esophageal mucosa.
Micro Pathology	Evidence of inflammation on biopsy; no malignant change noted.
Treatment	**Cessation of smoking**; elevation of head of bed; weight reduction; avoidance of fatty foods, coffee, chocolate, and alcohol; **H₂ receptor antagonists, proton pump inhibitors**, and **antacids** provide symptomatic relief; metoclopramide increases lower esophageal sphincter pressure and speeds gastric empty-ing, preventing reflux; surgery (e.g., Nissen fundoplication).
Discussion	The pathophysiology of gastroesophageal reflux disease (GERD) involves a sustained **decrease in LES tone** (caused by muscle weakness, scleroderma-like diseases, pregnancy, smoking, alcohol, or surgery), which allows reflux to occur. The extent of damage depends on the amount of refluxed material per episode, the frequency of episodes, the clearance rate by gravity and peristalsis, and the rate of neutralization of acids by salivary secretion. Chronic untreated GERD can lead to stricture forma-tion or columnar metaplasia of distal esophagus epithelium (BARRETT'S ESOPHAGUS), which predisposes to esophageal **adenocarcinoma**.

GASTROENTEROLOGY

ID/CC	A 50-year-old **Caucasian** male presents with progressively increasing **yellowing of the eyes** (JAUNDICE), a peculiar **skin rash**, and **palpitations**.
HPI	On directed questioning, he admits to having **decreased libido**. Three years ago he was diagnosed with **diabetes** and is on oral hypoglycemics. He smokes and drinks alcohol only occasionally, has never received a blood transfusion, and has no prior history of jaundice.
PE	Generalized **bronze discoloration** of skin; irregularly irregular pulse; icterus; loss of pubic and axillary hair; testicular atrophy; firm, nontender, nonpulsatile hepatomegaly.
Labs	Increased blood glucose; elevated LFTs; decreased serum testosterone and gonadotropins; **increased serum iron; decreased total iron-binding capacity; transferrin saturation > 80%; serum ferritin > 1000 μg/L (best screening method)**; desferrioxamine-chelatable urinary Fe excretion > 7.5 g Fe; **hepatic Fe quantitation > 100 μmol/g dry weight** (diagnostic). ECG: **atrial fibrillation**.
Imaging	CT, abdomen: diffusely increased liver density. Echo: **cardiomyopathy**.
Gross Pathology	Liver shows pigmentary cirrhosis.
Micro Pathology	Cirrhosis with abundant hemosiderin deposition in liver cells, Kupffer cells, and bile ducts.
Treatment	Repeated phlebotomies; monitor for development of **hepatoma** (due to increased risk); **screen first-degree relatives**.
Discussion	In idiopathic hemochromatosis, iron accumulates until the total body iron content reaches 50 g. The cause is a breakdown in the normal control of iron absorption from the GI tract; normally, the amount of iron accumulated inversely affects the GI mucosal absorption of both heme and nonheme iron. As iron overload progresses, iron that is ordinarily stored in the cells of the reticuloendothelial system is deposited in the liver, joints, gonads, pancreas, heart, and skin.
Atlas Links	⬚UCV1⬚ PG-P1-090, PM-P1-090

HEMOCHROMATOSIS

ID/CC	A 50-year-old male with a history of **alcoholism** is unresponsive to stimuli when brought by a neighbor to the emergency room.
HPI	His neighbor states that he had **vomited blood** (HEMATEMESIS) three months ago but had received no treatment. The neighbor also says that the patient got drunk three times a week for four years until approximately one year ago.
PE	Muscle wasting; **icteric sclera; spider angiomata** (due to increased levels of estrogen); nodular, **hard hepatomegaly; caput medusae**; loss of hair on chest and genitalia; **ascites**; gynecomastia; testicular atrophy; parotid enlargement; **flapping tremor of hands** (ASTERIXIS); **palmar erythema**; slight pitting edema in lower extremities.
Labs	CBC/PBS: slight thrombocytopenia; macrocytic anemia. Increased bilirubin; elevated serum transaminase and alkaline phosphatase; **low serum albumin** with increased globulins; **prolonged PT; high blood ammonia.**
Imaging	UGI: **esophageal varices**. EGD: esophageal varices confirmed. CT/US, abdomen: enlarged and fatty liver; tortuous, dilated variceal vessels.
Gross Pathology	Early: enlargement and fatty infiltration of liver; late: brownish discoloration, hardening, and atrophy of liver parenchyma.
Micro Pathology	Necrosis of normal hepatocytes; diffuse replacement with fibrous connective tissue and lymphocyte infiltrate; **regenerating nodules of liver lacking normal organization**; eosinophilic Mallory bodies; bile-congested ductules and proliferation of fibroblasts.
Treatment	**Discontinue alcohol**; supportive treatment of ascites, encephalopathy, variceal bleeding, and anemia.
Discussion	Hepatic cirrhosis is most commonly caused by alcohol; less commonly it is caused by biliary diseases, hepatitis B and C, Wilson's disease, and hemochromatosis. End-stage liver disease leads to liver failure, nutritional deficiencies, GI bleeding, and toxic ammonemia. There is also an increased risk of hepatocellular carcinoma.
Atlas Links	UCV1 PG-P1-091A, PG-P1-091B, PM-P1-091, H-P1-091 UCV2 IM1-034A, IM1-034B

GASTROENTEROLOGY

HEPATIC CIRRHOSIS

ID/CC A 56-year-old male with yellowing of the eyes and skin (due to **severe jaundice**) is brought to the ER in an **agitated state**.

HPI He has been passing black, tarry, foul-smelling stools (MELENA) and has exhibited a **reversal of sleep pattern** with **daytime sleepiness**. A few months ago he **vomited blood** (HEMATEMESIS) and was admitted to the hospital, at which time he was diagnosed with **alcoholic liver cirrhosis**.

PE VS: tachycardia; tachypnea; hypotension. PE: **lethargic and somnolent**; marked **icterus; feculent, fruity breath** (FETOR HEPATICUS); signs of chronic liver disease found; asterixis, dysarthria, and primitive reflexes (suck and snout) demonstrated; exaggerated deep tendon reflexes; **ascites; liver span reduced; splenomegaly**.

Labs LFTs markedly elevated (increased serum bilirubin, AST, and ALT; decreased serum albumin, reversed albumin-to-globulin ratio); alkaline phosphatase moderately elevated; prolonged PT. EEG: symmetric slowing; triphasic waves.

Imaging Endoscopy (during previous admission): **bleeding esophageal varices**.

Treatment **Eliminate precipitating factors** (such as GI bleeding, electrolyte imbalance, and infection); institute high-calorie and very **low protein diet; bowel cleansing** with **enemas; neomycin** and **lactulose** (induces diarrhea and clears the gut; alters bowel flora; and converts NH_3 to NH_4^+, which is less absorbable).

Discussion The cause of hepatic encephalopathy is multifactorial and includes **elevated concentrations of blood ammonia, short-chain fatty acids, false neurotransmitters**, decreased branched-chain amino acids, and a circulating substance that has properties similar to that of benzodiazepine agonists that potentiate the action of **GABA**.

ID/CC	A 40-year-old **male** presents with complaints of increasing **yellowness** of his eyes and skin, **darkly colored urine**, and loss of appetite.
HPI	He has no history of blood transfusions, contact with other jaundiced persons, or exposure to an epidemic of hepatitis in the neighborhood; the patient is a known **alcoholic**.
PE	Fever; **icterus**; parotid enlargement; **Dupuytren's contracture** in left index and little finger; **palmar erythema**; mildly **tender hepatomegaly**; no splenomegaly or ascites.
Labs	CBC: microcytic anemia; leukocytosis. Elevated serum bilirubin; **elevated AST and ALT** (AST > ALT, usually by a factor of two) (typically seen in alcoholic liver disease; in other parenchymal liver diseases, ALT is more elevated); increased alkaline phosphatase and γ-glutamyl-transferase (GGT); serologic markers negative for hepatitis A, B, and C; PT prolonged.
Imaging	US, abdomen: hepatomegaly with coarsened echo texture suggestive of hepatitis and fatty infiltration.
Gross Pathology	Enlarged liver with yellow and greasy surface (shrunken size with micronodular surface is seen in cirrhotic stage).
Micro Pathology	**Hepatocellular necrosis, neutrophilic infiltration, and alcoholic hyaline bodies** (MALLORY BODIES); some hepatocytes distended with fat, displacing nucleus to side; perivenular and sinusoidal fibrosis also seen.
Treatment	**Abstinence** is essential; nutritional support; colchicine tried with variable success.
Discussion	Liver diseases produced by excessive consumption of ethanol include fatty liver, alcoholic hepatitis, and cirrhosis; fatty change and, to an extent, alcoholic hepatitis may reverse fully with abstinence. Ten to fifteen percent of chronic alcoholics develop cirrhosis. The severity of alcoholic hepatitis can range from mild illness to fulminant hepatic failure.
Atlas Link	UCV1 PM-P1-093

HEPATITIS—ALCOHOLIC

ID/CC	A 65-year-old **alcoholic male** presents with right upper quadrant pain, **jaundice, anorexia**, and progressive **abdominal distention** of 2 months' duration; the distention has rapidly worsened over the past 10 days.
HPI	He also complains of **weight loss**. He has a **history of chronic hepatitis** (due to hepatitis B) but has no history of hematemesis, melena, hematochezia, or altered sensorium.
PE	Jaundice; **palmar erythema; spider angiomata** over upper abdomen; **loss of axillary and pubic hair; nodular hepatomegaly; free fluid in peritoneal cavity** (ASCITES); mildly enlarged spleen.
Labs	Increased direct bilirubin; **decreased serum albumin**; increased serum transaminase; mildly elevated alkaline phosphatase; **prolonged PT; markedly elevated serum α-fetoprotein (AFP)**; positive serum hepatitis B virus (HBsAg) surface antigen.
Imaging	US/CT: irregular **enhancing hepatic mass**; enlarged spleen; **enlarged portal vein; ascites**. Angio: **hypervascularity** of hepatic mass.
Gross Pathology	Hepatomegaly with single bile-stained lobulated hepatic mass impinging into portal triad.
Micro Pathology	Ascitic fluid cytology is hemorrhagic and reveals presence of malignant cells; liver biopsy reveals macronodular **cirrhosis** and hepatocytes that grow in columns with three possible patterns: trabecular, acinar, and pseudoglandular.
Treatment	Tumor embolization; chemotherapy; consider surgical resection depending on stage.
Discussion	Hepatocellular carcinoma is a malignant primary neoplasm of the liver. In the Western world, it **usually arises from a cirrhotic liver** and, wherever prevalent, is frequently associated with **hepatitis B** and hepatitis C infection. Other predisposing conditions include hemochromatosis, Wilson's disease, α_1-antitrypsin deficiency, alcoholic cirrhosis, and aflatoxin B1. It is spread by **hematogenous** and lymphatic dissemination, often to the lungs.

HEPATOCELLULAR CARCINOMA

ID/CC	A 50-year-old male with advanced **alcoholic cirrhosis** develops **oliguria** and **abdominal distention**.
HPI	His **renal and electrolyte status** has been **steadily deteriorating**.
PE	VS: tachycardia. PE: jaundice; ascites; asterixis.
Labs	**BUN increases** disproportionately to **serum creatinine** (indicating prerenal azotemia); marked **increase in urinary osmolality**. UA: **no active sediment**; random urine sodium low.
Gross Pathology	Renal biopsy shows no abnormality.
Treatment	Reversal of renal failure can occur with successful liver transplantation. In contrast, survival on dialysis is generally limited by the severity of the hepatic failure. No proven drug therapy.
Discussion	Hepatorenal syndrome (HRS) refers to the development of acute renal failure in a patient with advanced hepatic disease. It is often caused by **fulminant hepatic failure, cirrhosis**, and, less frequently, a **metastatic tumor** or **severe alcoholic hepatitis**. HRS usually represents the end stage of a **reduction in renal perfusion** induced by increasingly severe hepatic injury. It carries a **high mortality**.

HEPATORENAL SYNDROME

ID/CC	A 65-year-old male with **unresectable carcinoma of the sigmoid colon** is evaluated for **hepatomegaly** that was detected on a follow-up exam.
HPI	The patient is undergoing chemotherapy and underwent palliative surgery 1 month ago.
PE	Marked **pallor; large nodular liver palpable**; ascites (due to peritoneal seeding); colostomy bag noted.
Labs	**Markedly elevated carcinoembryonic antigen (CEA)** levels; **markedly raised alkaline phosphatase**; other LFTs normal.
Imaging	CT/US, abdomen: multiple enhancing hepatic nodules. Sigmoidoscopy: infiltrating **"napkin-ring"** growth in sigmoid colon.
Gross Pathology	On autopsy, multiple nodules noted, some with central necrosis (due to insufficient vascular supply).
Treatment	Supportive management; consider RF ablation for solitary metastasis.
Discussion	Liver metastases are more common than primary tumors of the liver. The most common tumors that metastasize to the liver are colon, gastric, pancreatic, breast, and lung carcinomas.
Atlas Link	⬜Ⓤ︎Ⓒ︎Ⓥ︎①⬜ PG-P1-096

ID/CC	A 34-year-old **alcoholic** male complains of sudden-onset, unrelenting **midepigastric pain radiating to the lower thoracic spine**.
HPI	He also complains of associated **anorexia, nausea**, and **vomiting**. The pain becomes worse when he is supine.
PE	VS: **hypotension; tachycardia**. PE: pale, sweaty; in severe distress; **periumbilical ecchymoses** (CULLEN'S SIGN); **left flank ecchymosis** (GREY TURNER'S SIGN); marked **epigastric tenderness** and diffuse **rebound tenderness** but minimal rigidity; abdomen distended with markedly decreased bowel sounds.
Labs	CBC: leukocytosis. **Markedly elevated serum amylase** and **lipase; elevated glucose**; elevated SGOT and LDH; **hypocalcemia**. ABGs: hypoxemia.
Imaging	CXR/KUB: no free air under diaphragm; abrupt termination of gaseous transverse colon at splenic flexure (COLON CUTOFF SIGN); distended loop of bowel in proximal jejunum (SENTINEL LOOP). CT, abdomen: enlargement and **inhomogeneity** of pancreas; **streaky peripancreatic inflammation**.
Gross Pathology	Autopsy: pancreas reveals pasty white foci of **fat necrosis, hemorrhage,** and cystic cavitation.
Micro Pathology	Edema of connective tissue, polymorphonuclear infiltration, hemorrhage and necrosis of pancreatic acini; fat necrosis · appears as pale blue amorphous foci where adipocyte membranes are dissolved.
Treatment	**"Rest" the pancreas** (analgesics, IV fluids, no oral intake, nasogastric suction).
Discussion	**Gallstones** and **alcohol abuse** are etiologic factors in 90% of patients with acute pancreatitis. Gallstones are thought to cause pancreatitis by **transient obstruction at the ampulla of Vater**, which leads to increased pancreatic ductal pressure. Other causes include infections (e.g., mumps), hereditary pancreatitis, shock, acute ischemia, hypercalcemia, hypertriglyceridemia, and drugs (e.g., thiazides, sulfonamides). Complications include DIC, **shock**, ARDS, hypocalcemia, acute renal failure, and pancreatic pseudocyst.

GASTROENTEROLOGY

PANCREATITIS—ACUTE

ID/CC	A 24-year-old white female complains of **crampy abdominal pain**, inability to pass flatus, abdominal distention, nausea, and vomiting.
HPI	After lack of improvement with 24 hours of nasogastric-tube suction and IV fluid, she underwent laparotomy to relieve **bowel obstruction** (due to a large hamartoma).
PE	**Hyperpigmented macules** on **lips** and **buccal mucosa** and on palms, fingers, and toes; **multiple hamartomatous growths** palpated **throughout GI tract**.
Labs	CBC/PBS: **microcytic, hypochromic anemia** (due to moderate GI bleeding). **Positive stool guaiac** test.
Imaging	UGI/SBFT/BE: acute small bowel obstruction; multiple **polypoid growths** of jejunum, ileum, and colon.
Gross Pathology	Pedunculated nodules up to 2 cm in size in stomach, duodenum, jejunum, ileum, and colon.
Micro Pathology	**Increased melanin deposition in buccal mucosa and lips**; hamartomatous lesions rarely undergo malignant transformation; smooth muscle and connective tissue extend into the pedunculated polyps and form an arborizing network.
Treatment	Periodic surveillance; consider endoscopic removal of all polyps; treat complications such as **obstruction, intussusception, and bleeding**.
Discussion	Peutz–Jeghers syndrome is **autosomal dominant** and is one type of hereditary familial polyposis syndrome. Polyps are hamartomas with **low malignant potential**, so resection is performed only if polyps are symptomatic. The condition is associated with an **increased risk of extraintestinal cancer** (e.g., pancreas, breast, lung, ovary, uterus).

ID/CC	A **36-year-old** white **female** complains of dizziness, fatigue, weight loss, and **difficulty swallowing** solid food (DYSPHAGIA).
HPI	She has been concerned about a recent **craving for ice and clay** (PICA). She reports no nausea/vomiting or hematemesis/ melena.
PE	VS: tachycardia. PE: pale skin and mucous membranes; **spoon-shaped nails** (KOILONYCHIA); **smooth, shiny red tongue** (GLOSSITIS); stomatitis.
Labs	CBC/PBS: **microcytic, hypochromic anemia. Low serum iron**.
Imaging	UGI: thin membranes of squamous mucosa typically in mid- or upper esophagus (ESOPHAGEAL WEBBING).
Gross Pathology	Postcricoid esophageal concentric web.
Treatment	Esophageal dilatation; supplemental iron.
Discussion	Also called Paterson–Kelly syndrome, Plummer–Vinson syndrome is associated with an **increased risk of esophageal cancer**.

PLUMMER–VINSON SYNDROME

GASTROENTEROLOGY

ID/CC   A 55-year-old **woman** presents with increasing yellowing of the eyes (JAUNDICE), fatigue, and **chronic itching**.

HPI   She also has **rheumatoid arthritis and chronic thyroiditis**. She has no prior history of jaundice, does not drink alcohol, and has never received a blood transfusion.

PE   **Icterus**; numerous scratch marks and excoriations on the skin; xanthomas and **xanthelasma**; hepatomegaly, splenomegaly, and no ascites; rheumatoid joint deformities and goiter (due to chronic thyroiditis).

Labs   Raised ESR; **markedly elevated alkaline phosphatase**; mildly elevated direct bilirubin and aminotransferases; **elevated serum cholesterol** (> 300 mg/dL); high titers of serum **antimitochondrial antibody**.

Imaging   US, abdomen: hepatomegaly and splenomegaly.

Gross Pathology   Dark green, enlarged liver (in late stages, liver shows cirrhosis that cannot be distinguished from other causes).

Micro Pathology   Bile duct destruction with lymphocytic-plasmacytic infiltration of portal areas; **periportal epithelioid granuloma formation** and portal scarring with linking of portal tracts; periportal bile stasis noted (in advanced cases, cirrhosis may be found).

Treatment   Cholestyramine to control pruritus; immunosuppression; liver transplantation is the only definitive treatment.

Discussion   Primary biliary cirrhosis is a chronic liver disease of probable **autoimmune** etiology that occurs primarily in **middle-aged women** and is characterized by **nonsuppurative obliterative cholangitis that progresses to cirrhosis**; it is associated with other autoimmune diseases in 85% of cases. Complications include cirrhosis and portal hypertension, malabsorption due to steatorrhea, and osteoporosis due to malabsorption of vitamin D and calcium.

Atlas Link   UCV2 IM1-039

ID/CC	A 60-year-old male presents with complaints of **fever, generalized abdominal pain, persistent bloody diarrhea, and increasing rectal pain**.
HPI	He was diagnosed with ulcerative colitis several years ago and had been treated with sulfasalazine and prednisone for intermittent exacerbations.
PE	VS: fever (39.9°C); tachycardia (HR 120); mild hypotension (BP 88/50). PE: **toxic-looking patient**; pallor noted; abdominal exam reveals **generalized tenderness** and **reduced bowel sounds**.
Labs	CBC: normocytic, normochromic anemia. RBCs, pus, and epithelial cells seen on stool exam.
Imaging	XR, abdomen (including cross-table lateral): **moderate dilatation** of **descending colon; thickened colonic wall** (due to wall edema); no evidence of intestinal perforation. CT, abdomen: no evidence of diverticular abscesses. Barium enema is contraindicated due to risk of perforation.
Gross Pathology	Moderate dilatation of colon; rectal mucosa friable and swollen; complete loss of mucosal folds.
Micro Pathology	Diffuse mononuclear infiltrate in lamina propria with neutrophils, mast cells, and eosinophils.
Treatment	**Bowel decompression** with nasogastric suction; fluid and electrolyte replacement; **parenteral antibiotics** to prevent sepsis; corticosteroids may be indicated to suppress inflammatory reaction in gut; **surgical colectomy** if immediate medical measures fail.
Discussion	Toxic megacolon results from complete shutdown of colonic neuromuscular function due to inflammation of the **myenteric neural plexus**. It may be seen as a complication of Crohn's disease, **ischemic colitis, pseudomembranous colitis**, and **ulcerative colitis**.

TOXIC MEGACOLON

ID/CC A 31-year-old male complains of having more than five bowel movements a day together with **cramping abdominal pain** and **tenesmus**.

HPI The patient adds that his stools consist of watery or pasty material with **mucus** and gross quantities of **blood**. He also complains of intermittent fatigue, fever, and an increased need for sleep.

PE VS: mild fever. PE: localized tenderness over distal colon.

Labs CBC: anemia; leukocytosis; hypoalbuminemia. Elevated ESR; stool exam reveals **no parasites; no bacterial pathogen** isolated in culture.

Imaging BE: early mucosal granularity; later, rigidity and **loss of haustrations** ("LEAD PIPE"), with ragged ulcerated mucosa and ulcerations. Colonoscopy: **mucosal erythema and granularity** with hemorrhaging and **inflammatory pseudopolyps**.

Gross Pathology Scarring and coarse, granular mucosal surface indicating presence of microulcerations; mucosal surface is friable; **lesions are continuous** from anal to oral direction.

Micro Pathology Increased numbers of lymphocytes, plasma cells, and PMNs; atrophy of mucosal glands and presence of PMNs in crypts of Lieberkühn (often called crypt abscesses); inflammatory changes confined to mucosa and submucosa.

Treatment Antidiarrheal drugs; sulfasalazine, 5-ASA preparations; glucocorticoids; cyclosporine for severe colitis; surgery if indicated (total proctocolectomy is curative).

Discussion Patients with ulcerative colitis are at **increased risk for colon cancer**. Factors favoring the development of colon cancer in ulcerative colitis are the duration of disease for 8 years or longer, involvement of the entire colon, continuous clinical activity, and, possibly, a severe initial attack. It is routinely advised that patients undergo regular surveillance that includes colonoscopy and an examination of multiple biopsies for dysplastic changes or frank cancer. Major complications include toxic megacolon and massive intestinal hemorrhage with shock and sepsis. Extraintestinal manifestations may include arthritis, erythema nodosum, ankylosing spondylitis, and sclerosing cholangitis.

Atlas Links ⬛UCVI⬛ PM-P1-102A, PG-P1-102, PM-P1-102B

ULCERATIVE COLITIS

ID/CC	A 43-year-old white male complains of severe **burning epigastric pain** and **diarrhea** of 2 years' duration that has been refractory to medical management.
HPI	The pain awakens him early in the morning, is accompanied by nausea and vomiting, increases with coffee consumption, and also appears 2 to 3 hours after meals. Three days ago, he also noticed **black stools**.
PE	Slight discomfort on epigastric palpation but no signs of peritoneal irritation; pale skin and mucous membranes; **occult blood** on digital rectal exam.
Labs	Fasting **serum gastrin markedly increased; increased gastric acid output** (HYPERCHLORHYDRIA) (due to elevated gastrin).
Imaging	CT/MR/Angio: small lesion in pancreas, difficult to localize. UGI/SBFT: atypical ulcers; gastric fold thickening.
Gross Pathology	**Ulcers in uncommon places** in esophagus, duodenum, and jejunum (due to excessive gastrin secretion); **gastrinoma** (commonly in pancreas or duodenum).
Micro Pathology	Usually originate from **delta cells** of pancreas; original lesion may be adenoma, hyperplasia, or carcinoma; hyperplasia of antral gastrin-producing cells.
Treatment	High-dose omeprazole; surgical resection if well localized and no metastases; gastrectomy; vagotomy.
Discussion	Zollinger–Ellison syndrome causes painful chronic diarrhea (vs. intestinal parasites, carcinoid syndrome, ulcerative colitis); roughly half may be malignant. It is associated with **multiple endocrine neoplasia (MEN) type I** (WERMER'S SYNDROME).
Atlas Links	UCV1 **PM-P1-103** UCV2 MC-112

ZOLLINGER–ELLISON SYNDROME

A 5-year-old otter cub, complaint of ... increasing gastric pain and dilation of ... ... the anterior portion of the ... ... gastric mucosal damage, and ...

MRI The pathologic agent in the gastric ... ...
... ...
... ...

CE ... ...
... ...
... ...

US ... ...
... ...

Imaging ... ...
... ...

Gross Pathology Ulcers in uncommon places in ... ...
... ...
... ...

Micro Pathology ... ...
... ...
... ...

Treatment ... ...
... ...

Discussion Zollinger-Ellison syndrome ... ...
... ...
... ...
... neoplasia (MEN) type 1 ... ...

Also cited ... ...

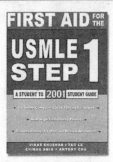
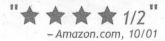
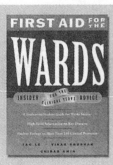
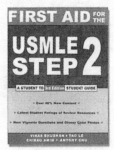
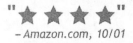

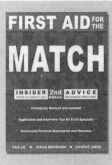